BIRTHING LIBERATION

BIRTHING LIBERATION

How
Reproductive
Justice Can
Set Us Free

SABIA WADE

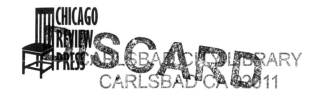

CHICAGO
REVIEW
PRESS

Copyright © 2023 by Sabia Wade
Foreword © 2023 by Michelle Phillips
All rights reserved
Published by Chicago Review Press Incorporated
814 North Franklin Street
Chicago, Illinois 60610
ISBN 978-1-64160-796-4

Library of Congress Control Number: 2022946315

Hand lettering: Sadie Teper
Typesetting: Nord Compo

Printed in the United States of America
5 4 3 2 1

To my sassy-ass maternal lineage
that I've had the blessing of witnessing
and learning from in this life:

My great-great-grandmother, **Gladys Hardy**,

My great-grandmother, **Ardel King**,

My grandmother, **Mariam Hardy**,

My mother, **La'Shayla King**.

I hope this book assists with our intergenerational healing
as much as I've healed from the strength and love
I've gathered from all of you.

Gentle black women
While being hated, yet teaching love
Being scorned, yet teaching respect
Being humiliated and teaching Compassion.

—Margaret Burroughs,
"Homage to Black Madonnas"

CONTENTS

FOREWORD

———

MANY PEOPLE ARE talking about liberation these days. I truly believe that the collective consciousness is on its way to understanding the full extent of what liberation means and what it takes to achieve it. We're not there yet. At the root, liberation starts with grief.

Before we can heal, enact any change in ourselves or the world, mobilize any calls to action, or push legislation or policy for reproductive justice, we must fully understand, know intimately, acknowledge, and grieve all the ways in which we are not free.

Grief is a normal and expected reaction to loss, change, and transition. Grief is a feeling that happens in our bodies and is fleshy, messy, and tactile—just like birth. Allowing ourselves to fully grieve everybody who has died due to the broken perinatal system becomes our love standing up. When we allow ourselves to begin at this beginning, we can genuinely do the work of becoming free.

Our choices can also set us free. If I had to choose a voice to walk me through the trenches toward reproductive justice at this unprecedented time, it would be the voice of Sabia Wade, the Black Doula.

I spoke with Sabia before writing a third version of this foreword. I had to know who Reena was, and it turns out she is an amalgam of all Sabia's clients and all Sabia's students' clients.

In our conversation, we remembered grief as the starting point in this work. It was grief that had driven Sabia to write in the first place. Grief is a familiar void I notice as a spiritual care practitioner. I kept asking myself what a doula would have done to support this family in making sense of their risk, grief, loss, death, and love. What would Sabia Wade, the Black Doula, do? Who was Reena to us? We already know this isn't even her name. And, yet, Reena is us, and she is ours.

It can be hard to conceptualize grief through the lens of popular grief theorists like Elizabeth Kübler-Ross. It can be problematic for Black folks, and Kübler-Ross created her stages of grief for individuals going through their own end-of-life processes. Her work does not touch on the systematic oppression and the resulting intergenerational trauma that makes for the deep complexity of Black bereavement. And so much more is emerging.

The wages of sin are death. If we look at sin as our transgressions, our mistakes, and the ways we miss the mark in providing holistic perinatal care to the least among us, those most marginalized and brutalized in this system, we pay the highest cost inside a broken system designed to fail us—Black birthers, Black babies, Black bodies.

If you are not holding grief and death in the work of birth, you aren't doing it right. Centered at the veil between this life and the next is birth. I'm willing to bet that the average birth professional or reproductive justice advocate did not get into this work because they wanted to do death care, and yet, here we are.

Sabia has started this journey for us.

Sabia is more than a new client and the work toward liberation is ever evolving. Bravery allows her to start this journey knowing she can't purchase a return ticket.

In this book, she unwinds what we know to be true about the current state of the Black birthing experience in this country, contextualizes how we got here, and visions us toward a wholly embodied birthing liberation. Sabia articulates the historical imprint of violence, brutality, trauma, and the continued systemic oppression of birth in the United States, but she goes deeper to where this all lands: on our bodies, the sanctuary of our freedom.

Sabia's work will stand as a guide to help us heal and free ourselves of the cloak of oppression because we already are. I hope you cry, shout, develop curricula, teach courses, lead workshops and book groups, plan podcasts, write talks, craft speeches, conjure spells, spark revolutions, and birth your own liberation, all with underlined and well-worn copies of this book. I pray you drink the sometimes-bitter words as good medicine and love it as I already do.

We also know the journey will be different when we allow ourselves to grieve first—attending to the life and the living, the death and the dying *in the room where it happens.*

Sabia's soul is on that much deeper journey; she's on her way to attend to the risk, grief, loss, death, and love. And if I know Sabia, and I believe I do, she'll come back for us.

Stay attuned.

Michelle Phillips, the Liberation Strategist

ACKNOWLEDGMENTS

FIRST AND FOREMOST, I want to acknowledge and thank all of the people, visible and hidden, doing reproductive justice work and all forms of activism. This work ain't easy! It takes so much energy, time, and dedication to continue moving through this work and through this world. I thank you for being in community with me, teaching me about this work and myself, loving me through my mistakes, and showing up for all the folks in our communities who do not always have the ability to show up for themselves. You are appreciated!

Thank you to Nikki Van De Car, my book coach, for assisting me in writing the literal first words for this book. Thank you, Laura Lee Mattingly, my book agent, for not only believing in my vision but also always aiming to keep it true to its purpose. Thank you to Kara Rota and Chicago Review Press, my editor and publisher, for getting it and assisting me in the heavy lifting of writing. To all of y'all, I know I constantly questioned why the hell I decided to write this book, but I get it now!

To all my family and friends who have supported me through the ups and downs of writing this treasure, I love all of you and I'm so grateful for your patience as I moved through this process, sometimes happy and sometimes overwhelmed. I can't possibly name all of you, but to name a few: Venice, Jacob, Elijah, Jenna, Dashawne, Davina, Euni, and Jen Mayer!

To my ancestors: PHEW! Your life, your work, your suffering, and your joy has not been in vain. This book is all of yours too!

Lastly, shout-out to my therapist for keeping me above water for the last couple of years because BABYYYYY, IT'S BEEN A ROUGH ONE!

Love you all, and I'm more than blessed to receive all your love and support!

I'm living the life of my dreams!

INTRODUCTION

———

WE ALL KNOW the stats. The perinatal mortality rate for Black birthing people is three to four times higher than it is for white patients (and this percentage goes up even more in some spaces). The data is so overwhelming, and so terrible, that it can seem impossible to overcome. The statistics alone are traumatizing. And this is just one out of countless examples of racism as a national health crisis. We often say that racism comes from society and "the system," and while that may be true, it can give us permission to see it as a problem that is unsolvable—certainly not by any single individual. But the truth is that we do have agency, and in fact each of us has a responsibility to unlearn our own racialized trauma and bias. Racism is upheld by people, and it is only when people do the work that we can finally liberate ourselves from it.

We hear that phrase a lot: "do the work." What does it mean, exactly? Reading about racism, hashtagging Black Lives Matter, sending money—that is not doing the work. We call it work because it isn't easy, and it requires moving beyond the cognitive experience and deconstructing how racism lives in your own body. When we logically approach our racism, we skip implicit bias, the racism that we aren't aware of but that is living within our bodies nonetheless.

Why Birthing Liberation

So how do we do the work? We start by learning about the past and understanding how our history has created our present reality. When we look at present-day gynecology, we think of all the lifesaving practices that have been created, but we might not know that these specific tools and techniques were developed through experimentation on and abuse against Black bodies. We don't recall how Black Granny midwives were leading communal reproductive health until they were pushed aside by white male doctors, thereby denying Black birthing people reproductive care. Even now, when we look at these horrifying statistics, we know that they are intimately related to the shortage of Black midwives and doulas, and that Black birthing people still are not getting the support they deserve and need. Black perinatal mortality statistics have not improved in the past thirty years. In fact, recent research published by Neel Shah, assistant professor of obstetrics, gynecology, and reproductive biology at Harvard Medical School, shows that BIPOC parents have higher rates than those in non-BIPOC communities when it comes to the percentage of babies born preterm or with low birth weight.* Even with increasing talk of "raising awareness," protests, and the many calls to action, nothing is actually changing for Black people. We are still being shot and killed without cause, we are still dying during childbirth from avoidable complications that would not and do not cause the deaths of white birthing people and white infants, and Black parents are still left questioning the potential for their

---

* National Academies of Sciences, Engineering, and Medicine, *Birth Settings in America: Outcomes, Quality, Access, and Choice* (Washington, DC: The National Academies Press, 2020), 26, https://doi.org/10.17226/25636.

children to have full, happy, long lives without the sometimes deadly interruption of racism.

And nothing will change unless we address the internal experience, unless we dive deeper into a more embodied understanding of the history and present experience of racism and the ongoing racial trauma we all experience—and how to heal it within ourselves. *Birthing Liberation* explains the history of racism and its impact on our present day as well as the perinatal and infant mortality crisis currently plaguing the Black community. *Birthing Liberation* teaches us, not only how to understand our own trauma resulting from racism and our current systems, but also how to begin to heal it through somatic practices, journaling, and internal awareness, helping the reader access tools for healing that we already carry within ourselves. The ability to understand the past can help us change the future and help us understand how we embody racism on a somatic level, beyond the cognitive experience. *Birthing Liberation* explains exactly what racial trauma is, discusses how it is experienced by both Black and white people, and explores why white people feel so much discomfort and emotion in conversations about race, as well as providing tools to move through discomfort and into positive impact and change.

About the Author

I began my journey into the birth world in 2015 when I became a volunteer full-spectrum doula for the Prison Birth Project (PBP) based in Chicopee, Massachusetts, after being a certified nursing assistant and realizing the many inequities facing marginalized communities in the medical system. Prior to taking the step to become a doula, I was working in a Philadelphia hospital system. I started to question if I wanted to be a nurse because it was the natural next step after being a nursing assistant for some years or if I truly felt becoming an RN was a part of my individual path and personal fulfillment. I had also become aware of

doulas at this time because of the work being done by doulas in Philadelphia communities. I was interested in learning more about doulas,
especially because of their autonomy and the gaps they were filling in
community care, but I didn't have the time to dive deeper into doula
care. During that period of internal questioning, I was having visceral
reactions to the experience of being in a system that seemed to prioritize
budgets over people, especially if those people weren't white, male, and
financially stable. The stress of this internal battle came to a peak when
my heart began to race uncontrollably (between 160 and 180 beats per
minute while sitting) during a shift and would not decrease. I was sent
to the emergency room, monitored for hours, and sent home without
a clear diagnosis or reason for my discomfort and racing heart. In the
following weeks, I was unable to return to work and was battling with
a racing and unstable heart rate, being light-headed most of the time,
and only finding relief when I laid down. I went to see a cardiologist
(a non-BIPOC male) feeling excited about *finally* getting the special-
ized care I needed. The result of that appointment was a doctor who
patronizingly told me I was fine and probably just dehydrated, even
after I shared how debilitated I was. To be honest, that was my first
experience of needing care and realizing my skin color may have been
a factor in the lack of care I received. I can still feel the disappointment
and heaviness in my body that came with being dismissed and feeling
helpless. However, there was a gift that came from this experience: my
decision to move to Massachusetts and become a full-spectrum doula.
I realized becoming an RN was not a part of my path and the only way
to jump into doula work was to go all the way, even with the fear I had
about going on a path that didn't have a clear road, and work with a
community that many never thought or really cared about.

As a volunteer for PBP for two years, I served incarcerated and
formerly incarcerated birthing people dealing with substance abuse disorder. During that time, I was also introduced to the concept and lifestyle of reproductive justice by the founder of PBP, Marianne Bullock.

Reproductive justice changed the way I saw my world, especially as I began to understand that everything, from the water we drink to the ways that Black and Indigenous birthing bodies are undervalued, is intrinsically connected to reproductive justice. As I was diving into this world of reproductive justice and doula work, I was assigned to my first doula client. She was expecting her first child and living in a recovery home after spending some time in jail. She wasn't feeling very supported by her family or the father of her child, and also was holding on to a high amount of shame over her substance abuse history. At the same time as I was connecting with my first client, I was experiencing intense back pain and pressure and pain at the bottom of my ribs. The pain was unfamiliar and continued to get worse and relentless as days passed. As I was navigating my own pain, I also supported my client with an in-home maternity photoshoot and showing up at a couple unexpected hospital visits. I was finally feeling aligned with the work I was doing, but I was also realizing that it was time to address the physical pain I was now enduring constantly.

After getting off my day job, I decided to go to urgent care to be seen for my pain in hopes of gaining some clarity because I knew without hesitation that something was not right. I was seen by a doctor (again, a non-BIPOC male) for all of five minutes. He did not lay a hand on me, even though I was complaining of pain in and around my abdomen. He told me I most likely had a kidney stone, even though I had no former history of kidney issues in my twenty-seven years of life, and prescribed pain medication. Two days later there was no improvement, so I went to a different urgent care center hoping a different location and doctor would improve my experience. I was seen by a doctor (another non-BIPOC male), and once again the level of care was subpar—no palpation or touch to my abdomen at all, even with my very specific complaints and knowledge about my body. This time I was diagnosed with gallbladder stones and given more medication. After two more additional days, I wasn't able to be seen by my primary doctor but was able to be seen by a doctor (an Indian male) in the practice. This time, the doctor listened to what I was experiencing, palpitated my abdomen, and sent me for additional testing. A couple short days later, I was officially diagnosed with a uterine fibroid that was decreasing the size of my bladder and my rectum and pushing against my spine. Without treatment, I was heading toward increased pain and abdominal issues.

On January 1, 2016, I attended my first birth, and it was a complicated, magical, and unforgettable experience. My client was formerly incarcerated and in substance abuse recovery. We had built a beautiful relationship where she could be forthcoming with me in ways she couldn't even with people who were close to her. She had a successful vaginal delivery, and I remember thinking nothing could be more beautiful than birth. I also remember feeling the weight of holding all the complexities that came with her experience and wondering how others with complex realities were moving through parenthood without the support of a doula.

On January 5, 2016, I had an open abdominal surgery to remove the uterine fibroid, and the process was necessary, painful, and so complicated. I could tell you more about how I was fired from my employment and how I sued for race and disability discrimination, was denied unemployment, and after an appeal, was ultimately offered it, while also having complications and many emergency room visits that later resulted in postsurgical fibromyalgia and chronic pelvic pain conditions. Through all these experiences I constantly thought about how other people, especially Black people, were treated in similar situations. I had a medical background, knew my options, and advocated for myself relentlessly, but it took a third visit in one week to a physician of color to finally get the care I needed. The combination of my personal experience and volunteer experience solidified my path to becoming a lifelong advocate of reproductive justice for all.

At the end of 2016, I experienced my second abdominal surgery to deal with scar tissue connecting my bowel to my uterus. I was fortunate to work with a practice of doctors that understood my pain was life altering and would only continue to diminish my quality of life. At that time, I even contemplated having a hysterectomy at the age of twenty-eight. I had a physician who was fully supportive but also created a successful alternative plan to avoid the hysterectomy. Some studies show that Black patients receive hysterectomies at rates that are three times higher than white patients, and many of these hysterectomies are unnecessary and cause additional long-term issues, such as menopausal symptoms, depression, and even poorer cardiac health. In the South this statistic is even more astonishing—"up to 90% of hysterectomies among Black patients at rural hospitals occur in the region."[*] Once I was finally cleared by my gynecologist at the beginning of 2017, I decided to move to San Diego, California, partially because I hate snow but also because I knew I wanted to be a full-time doula eventually and my research showed San Diego was full of doula opportunities. I soon learned that the opportunities for Black, Indigenous, and people of color (BIPOC) doulas and non-BIPOC doulas were different and imbalanced. In 2018 I quit my job and became a full-time doula and then experienced racism and discrimination from non-BIPOC birthing people and birth workers. I experienced non-BIPOC high-earning doulas only sending me free and low-cost client opportunities, as if I didn't have bills to pay myself. I also experienced clients of other doulas requesting me to fill in for them urgently and ignoring me when they realized I was Black, along with many other racist and insulting experiences. That same year, I began my nonprofit, For the Village, the only community doula organization centering Black birthing people and their children in San Diego. I created For the Village to focus

---

[*] Amy Yurkanin, "Why Do Black Women Get More Hysterectomies in the South?," Center for Health Journalism, February 1, 2022, https://centerforhealthjournalism .org/2022/01/28/why-do-black-women-get-more-hysterectomies-south.

on community care with an emphasis on Black birthing people who deserved access to doula care, and who also deserved a space that was not connected to any of the hospital systems and was specially built to truly serve community members without bias or fear. I was also being approached by BIPOC community members wanting to serve their community as a doula but continuously met with barriers to training. For the Village supports community members interested in becoming doulas by providing a free full-spectrum doula training and paying them for their services while providing free doula services to low-income families and to all Black birthing people, who according to current research, are at a higher risk of having a negative birth outcome regardless of their income level or social identities.

In 2019 I officially shifted my brand from Doula Sabia to the Black Doula and began my birth worker training organization, Birthing Advocacy Doula Trainings (BADT). I was surprisingly and consistently being asked to mentor and train doulas, but I couldn't find a training organization that I felt aligned with. The organizations I encountered at the time seemed to always speak about BIPOC and marginalized groups as the "others" and were surprisingly either uninterested in or unaware of reproductive justice, disparities, and all the issues that were so central to my interest in becoming a doula. I wanted to train in a space that centered my experiences, and it seemed others were looking for this space as well—so I decided to create it. BADT not only trains our students to serve their clients using the best practices available, but we also provide them with a wide perspective of disparities, inequalities, policies, and rights, and prepare them to be active partners in the movement to change birth and reproductive health culture locally, nationally, and globally. We have trained over eight thousand students all over the world.

In 2019 I also offered my first free webinar, titled "Racism & Privilege in Birth Work," as a preview to a BADT course of the same name. With one share I had hundreds of birth workers wanting to take part in this discussion and many more starting to follow my work because of the course. Within a few months, I expanded the course into an eight-hour, two-day, in-person offering that successfully sold out in many cities, including Seattle, Boston, and San Diego. People attending this course ranged from executive directors in hospital systems to doulas. All were seeking a similar understanding of how racism and privilege greatly affected birth work and what their personal responsibility in this collective crisis was. I witnessed many emotions and traumas, as well as the desire to be better, in both BIPOC and non-BIPOC people. There were many tears, hugs, fits of rage, and conversations—and those moments further motivated me to write this book. Currently, I continue to teach many birth workers from both hospital and out-of-hospital backgrounds, as well as in colleges, therapy practices, corporate companies, and other locations, utilizing my course "Racism & Privilege in Birth Work" and teaching about related topics such as trauma-informed care and the importance of gender inclusion in all spaces.

Long before becoming a doula and finding my life path in reproductive justice, I was a Black person navigating the world, dealing with racism, microaggressions, and hearing about how often Black people are shot, how often they die in childbirth, and how often we suffer daily for no other reason than the color of our skin. I speak from my own experience with seeing a lack of true, sustainable, healing change from the people who claim they want a more equal world. My struggles and my internal process have made me anxious, depressed, and dissociated from my body . . . but the practice of somatic experience continually brings me back to myself. Becoming a student and consumer of somatic healing practices, and then fusing that with my work as a doula and educator, inspired me to bring all of the pieces of my life together to create a tool for revolution, a framework for how we can all achieve liberation.

Collective liberation is the idea that in order for us all to have equity in this world—equity meaning anything from the safety of birthing children to the ability to bring a baby home to a safe community (which is another form of reproductive justice)—we must all become liberated individuals. A liberated individual is someone who understands their own trauma, what they are good at, and what they need to work on, and who also understands that to shift power to those who are more marginalized and in turn less privileged, as well as unable to access power, does not make them smaller. On the contrary, it makes everyone bigger, better, and, more important, puts them on the continuous path of healing. Liberation does not mean that trauma will cease to exist. But it does mean that our trauma can exist and not overtake our right to live, love, and be in community with others, including those who may not always understand us. Liberation means you have the power to share power, to coexist and cocreate with others with the full awareness of yourself, including both the parts of yourself that are well-tuned and those that are still under construction. Collective liberation empowers us all.

The liberation of individuals creates liberated communities, which can serve as spaces of purpose, advocacy, and also healing. Liberated communities are necessary for sustainable power and action. These communities, as they join together, are how we can overcome the seemingly insurmountable challenges of societal and systemic change. Systemic change feels impossible, but when you break them down, systems are nothing more than broken and traumatized communities—and communities are made up of people. By achieving individual liberation and coming together as a liberated community, we can serve as a true model for equity and shared power, breaking through the trauma and barriers that have stood in the way of equality and true, lasting change.

Language is everything. Unless directly speaking to a particular community or making direct comparison, this book centers BIPOC people and their experiences by using the terms *BIPOC* as a way of describing Black, Indigenous, and people of color and *non-BIPOC* to describe white people. This shift in language is essential to decentering the non-BIPOC experience as the standard and the "right" or dominant way of existing and creates space for the many races, cultures, and identities that exist but are often ignored. This shift in language may feel difficult for some and disorienting for many, but I challenge you to use this language in your daily life and notice the changes and reactions in others as you normalize this language and approach to centering the most marginalized. I also want to invite folks not to say BIPOC when they are speaking to a particular community. For example, I will use Black when I mean Black, instead of the larger BIPOC category. Gender-neutral language—speaking and writing in a way that does not discriminate against a particular sex, social gender, or gender identity, and does not perpetuate gender stereotypes—is also a foundation of this book. Gender-neutral language provides an inclusive and trauma-informed approach that creates space for people to self-identify should they choose to disclose this information about themselves. Not only women have the ability to give birth, and not everyone who undergoes pregnancy and birth is a woman. In this book, I will use the term *birthing person*, and instead of saying maternal, I may say *parental* to be inclusive to all genders. In addition, I will be using the term *Black perinatal health* instead of Black maternal health because many people in these statistics have not been asked for their gender identity or haven't felt safe enough to share their gender identities, and these stats include more than Black cis women. I also would like to note that mainstream data typically uses the term perinatal for folks beginning at seven months into pregnancy, rather than for the entire duration. However, in this book, we will be expanding that definition to mean the same thing as maternal as there isn't currently a term that is inclusive of all birthing people. Remember, inclusive language is not exclusive. Finally, I want to remind you that language is nuanced, so feel empowered to use language that works for you when addressing yourself. This process is all about holding space for yourself, as much as for others.

BIPOC readers, *Birthing Liberation* is not just my book; it is our book. This book is inspired by the past we have survived and the present we are actively working in and through, as well as the future we are committed to creating. This book may bring up emotions of anger, sadness, and pure frustration. I advise you to take your time and care for yourself in whatever ways that call to you. That may look like talking to a friend, pausing and returning at a later date, taking time to rest, or leaning on your spiritual practice for comfort and support. This book will also celebrate you, remind you of your greatness, and often remind you to rest, recharge, and refocus. It is not only our job to do the work; this work is collective and will require just as much work from non-BIPOC people. I hope this book reminds you of that and gives you the permission you need to not only be the fixer but also to be cared for mentally, physically, emotionally, and spiritually. We deserve that and more.

Non-BIPOC readers, I want to be very clear about the request that is being made of you. You are not only being asked to believe in equality and equity. You are being asked to move beyond belief and into action. In other words, a white ally is aware of racism and discrimination as common issues that infiltrate all systems and create hardship for BIPOC people and privilege for non-BIPOC people. A white ally also wants equity for BIPOC people and may even speak about this desire in their circles, but their actions toward changing the direction of our current world are little to none, which means they are continuing to benefit from systemic oppression and racism. Becoming a white accomplice is the next step, and it is vital to create an equitable and safer world for all people, especially BIPOC people. A white accomplice puts their beliefs into action that is led by the BIPOC community. White saviorism, a non-BIPOC person aiming to liberate or rescue BIPOC people without the opinions and leadership of the BIPOC community, is not supportive in the commitment to being a white accomplice, nor are white tears without the ability to self-regulate and decenter the white experience. That is the lifelong work you must commit to and the only way we can move forward toward the future we all need, a future that liberates all of us.

Birthing Liberation creates a path to social and systemic change through the practice of learning oneself, with the understanding that to learn oneself is to have the tools to create the capacity for a lifetime of true and measurable action that can create real change. *Birthing Liberation* is a call to action for the reader, and more than that, it teaches them how to take action. Because the truth is, we can no longer sustain passive action. The ideal reader for this book is ready to confront their shadows, drop their ego, heal their trauma, and accept their responsibility and their impact on others. It is time to do more than post a black square, read a book written by a Black author, schedule or attend a diversity and inclusion training, and call that a good day's anti-racism work. Yes, this person is less obviously racist than someone with a Confederate flag in their yard . . . but that doesn't mean that they are doing the actual work—work that is not merely self-serving, work that can contribute to the safety of Black people. The audience for this book is ready to do more.

It is everyone's responsibility to take action. We must liberate ourselves so we can work to liberate everyone.

How to Read This Book

It is important and appreciated if you take your time reading this book. I will remind you of this as you move along in the book. This book should also be read in chronological order, as each section builds on the last. There will be exercises in this book that consist of a mix of breathing, journaling, and sitting still and with self; please take the time to complete these exercises or come back to them when you can before moving on. Connecting with yourself beyond reading and logical thinking is required for truly embodying this information. I suggest each reader create a space for themselves before reading this book. Get comfortable. Perhaps get a blanket and a cup of tea, or even find a private closet to hide away in as you go through these pages.

Also, feel free to take breaks at any point; welcome in movement, emotion, and anything else that comes to you. I highly recommend always having a pen and paper ready for you to jot down any exercise notes or thoughts that find their way to your mind. All these pieces are important to this process, and none of them are more important than the other. Lastly, any time you read this book, I suggest you open and close your reading time with a ritual of some kind. This ritual could include calling in your ancestors for support or reminding yourself that you are *in process*, that having big feelings is OK, and that perfection is not a requirement in this space. When closing out your time with this book, you can invite in any movement your body is asking for and bring one of the exercises into this book into your day, reinforcing your mind/body connection.

When opening this book, be sure to find a private, or mostly private, space and gather anything you may need during your time with it (pen, paper, water, blanket, etc.). Breathe in deeply through your nose and out your mouth three times while consciously dropping your shoulders and releasing any tension in your body. Say, "At this time, I give myself permission to turn off the world and turn into myself with the support of my ancestors and guides." Take a few more breaths and begin reading when you feel ready. To close out of your time with this book, close your eyes and feel any sensations and messages happening within your body. Follow those messages to move, stretch, vocalize yourself, or even to write any messages down. Say, "Thank you for supporting me through this journey, ancestors and guides. Throughout the day, I will carry the feeling of liberation, and I will practice this ongoing work through this exercise."

Again, these are only examples, and I trust you will find the opening and closing exercise that works best for you and your needs. Before you move on, I want to thank you for your bravery, dedication, and belief in me and this book. None of it goes unnoticed!

1

IN THE ROOM
WHERE IT HAPPENS

It's very hard being in this home and imagining her here with us. She never got to even meet him. She never got to see him. And she was just so thrilled about having him.

—Bruce McIntyre III, the partner of Amber Rose Isaac, a victim of Black perinatal health disparities who died during childbirth after not receiving adequate care

THE COMMON, HARMFUL interactions between care providers and BIPOC birthing people are more than just statistics. They are real, lived traumas, and it is the responsibility of privileged communities not experiencing this trauma to confront this truth by listening to the voices of the most vulnerable as closely as possible, to *experience* it as closely as possible. And so, in this chapter, I walk you through a scenario of a Black birthing mother. You will experience her perspective, her partner's perspective, and her mother's perspective, as well as the perspective of her care providers. Reading this story won't be easy, but this is a real trauma that happens every day. We can't look away from it, and we can't stop it if we don't understand it. I also invite you to get comfortable with the different type of learning that will be happening throughout this book. In order to move through this book, there is also a requirement to embody what you are learning by moving past the intellectual aspect of your mind and into the physical knowledge of your body as well. The combination of learning though your mind *and* body will create a bigger and deeper impact that is long term and requires you to not only connect but also to be with the information you are consuming.

Before we begin, notice what sensations you may be experiencing just at the thought of reading through this type of story. Did you start to feel nervous, anxious, angry, or even checked out? I welcome you to take a few slow, deep breaths right now, directing your breath toward those spaces in your body that may feel tension and even resistance. As you read this chapter, pause, breathe deeply, and let the information enter not just your mind but also your body. That is the difference between consuming information and integrating it into your very being. Only when we deeply experience things will we be able to move forward to make true change.

What Happened

Reena is a twenty-six-year-old Black cis woman. She is pregnant with her first child and is currently in day two of the birthing process at a local hospital in Atlanta, Georgia. Reena has felt well and balanced throughout her pregnancy and planned for a vaginal birth without any interventions. Unfortunately, her birth is not going the way she hoped. She is making progress, although not as quickly as her care providers would like. She eventually chose to have an epidural to assist with pain control. Reena is being supported by her mother, Hilary (a Black cis woman), and her partner, Jarrod (a Black cis man). Reena's care team consists of a nurse, Samantha (a non-BIPOC cis woman), and a doctor, Dr. Smith (a non-BIPOC cis man).

At 12:00 PM during the second day, thirty hours into Reena's labor, Dr. Smith comes into her room. He greets her, her mother, and her partner briefly, then proceeds to let them know that since Reena has been laboring for more than twenty-four hours, she should start to think about a cesarean section. He says that if the baby does not arrive within a few hours, it will become necessary. Jarrod wonders why a few more hours is the cutoff point, but he nods his head and doesn't ask any questions. Reena maintains eye contact with Dr. Smith but does not give any sign that she has fully understood what he has said.

Reena's mother, Hilary, stands up immediately and asks the doctor, "Why do you believe a cesarean section is the next step? She seems fine, and the baby hasn't shown any signs of stress." In an authoritative tone and upright posture, Dr. Smith explains that hospital policy is to perform a C-section for any patient that has not given birth within thirty-six hours. After Dr. Smith leaves the room, Hilary says she doesn't trust the hospital or the care providers and decides to take a break. She leaves the room to go get some fresh air.

After Hilary leaves, Reena and Jarrod talk about the possibility of a C-section. Both feel nervous about it but hope that the surgery will go well and that their medical staff will take care of them. The nurse, Samantha, comes in to get an update on Reena's vitals. Samantha is caring and supportive of Reena, but she is also distracted by the amount of charting she must complete. Samantha quickly gets a blood pressure reading on Reena. She smiles at Reena and lets her know her blood pressure is a little high, but that it's probably from the conversation about the possible C-section, so it's nothing to worry about.

Hilary comes back into the room, still talking about how she doesn't trust the medical system. She tells Reena a story she's told many times before, about her experience of Reena's birth. When Hilary went into labor, she checked into a hospital accompanied by her sister, April—at the time, a male partner wasn't allowed in the room. At first, things seemed to be going fine, but as her labor became more active, she needed more assistance from her non-BIPOC nurse—and she was met with dismissive responses. She was getting little to no information about what was happening with her own body, and her pain and fear were overwhelming her. When it was time to deliver Reena, the delivery team (all non-BIPOC) came into the room and began to set up. At this point, Hilary was understandably hysterical and looking for reassurance from the hospital staff. Instead, she was told to stop being dramatic, to quiet down, and to get into birthing position.

Hilary followed their directions and asked her sister to come closer to the bed so she could hold her hand for support. Hilary's nurse told her no and said, "I don't know why you people always have to be so dramatic." Hilary began pushing, but it didn't feel right. She asked the doctor to let her change positions, but he sternly told her no and threatened to take her to the OR if she did not deliver Reena soon. Hilary continued to push with all her might, even though her positioning was not ideal. At last she was able to successfully deliver Reena vaginally, and her daughter was absolutely perfect as Hilary held her in her arms.

But an hour after delivery, Hilary noticed that she was bleeding. She told the nurse, who checked her briefly, said that "bleeding is a part of the process," and left the room. A few minutes later, Hilary seemed out of sorts, so her sister checked her and found a large pool of blood growing under Hilary. April quickly alerted the nurse, who called out for assistance with an emergency. Hilary was experiencing postpartum hemorrhage, and if her sister had not checked on her bleeding at that exact time, she would have undoubtedly lost her life.

This is the first time Reena has heard this story, and it frightens her. She doesn't want to hear it right now, in the middle of her own labor, but she knows her mother needs to tell it. Listening to this under the circumstances exhausts her, and she goes to sleep. A couple of hours later, Reena wakes up and rings her nurse to let her know she has a headache that she is concerned about. She rarely ever gets headaches, and she feels like something could be wrong. The nurse assures her that she's fine, and that given the epidural and the amount of stress she is under, it's not surprising. Reena nods her head and goes back to resting. Jarrod and Hilary are exhausted but determined to stay by Reena's side no matter how long it takes. Around 6:00 PM, Dr. Smith comes into Reena's room, saying, "It's been a few hours, so I'm going to check your cervix for dilation." Reena has dilated an additional one to two centimeters, but the baby is still high in the pelvis, so the doctor directs Samantha to schedule a C-section in the next couple of hours. Reena begins to cry, saying she feels like a failure, and Dr. Smith quickly leaves the room.

Nurse Samantha's heart floods with compassion. She rushes to reassure Reena that she is not a failure and that these things just happen sometimes. Samantha has seen this happen time and again, and she believes that many of the C-sections she's witnessed were unnecessary. She leaves to speak privately to Dr. Smith, suggesting they wait a few more hours since Reena *is* progressing, even if it's not as quickly as they would prefer. She explains to Dr. Smith that since this is Reena's first child, it's likely her body just needs some time to get ready for delivery.

Dr. Smith doesn't look at her but keeps his eyes on the computer screen in front of him. He tells Samantha that he has made his final decision, and that his decision is what matters most. Samantha feels both angry and belittled, but she says, "Of course, sir, you know best," and follows his directions. She sees no other choice—this is her job.

Back in Reena's room, Hilary is very angry and tells Reena she is going to go speak to the doctor. Jarrod tells Hilary to calm down and asks her not to bring any additional tension to this already stressful situation. Reena tells them again that her headache is getting worse and she's not feeling well, so Jarrod timidly calls Samantha into the room. He tells her that Reena seems to be in a lot of pain and that she's not herself. Samantha assures him that she is just exhausted and stressed, but to make him feel better, she offers to take Reena's vitals. To her surprise, Reena's blood pressure is 180/120—hypertensive. She takes it again, and it reads the same. Hilary hits the emergency button on the wall, and Dr. Smith and several other staff members rush Reena to the OR for an emergency C-section. Because it's an emergency C-section, neither Hilary nor Jarrod is allowed into the operating room. Jarrod is at a loss for words, and Hilary is beyond furious. Reena is alone. Hilary and Jarrod wait in the empty hospital room in silence.

An hour later Dr. Smith returns to the hospital room. He tells them that Reena had a severe case of preeclampsia that progressed to eclampsia. Preeclampsia is a dangerous pregnancy complication that can cause high blood pressure and other harmful side effects. If it is not diagnosed and treated, it can progress to eclampsia, which can cause seizures and even death—which is what happened. In a monotone voice, Dr. Smith states that he was able to save the baby but, unfortunately, Reena did not make it through the procedure. Dr. Smith says he is sorry for their loss and quickly walks away, though Samantha stays present to support Jarrod and Hilary. Jarrod stands there in shock while Hilary collapses into his arms. Neither of them can understand how these care providers could have missed this diagnosis. How will they continue without Reena? Jarrod is now a widower and a single father. Hilary is now a childless mother, and Reena's baby, Tyler, a motherless child.

> Pause.
>
> Take a moment to somatically take in the details of Reena's story by absorbing the details of this story and listening to the messages your body is sending to you through sensations that may feel like buzzing, heaviness, sharpness, or even literal pain in parts of your body. Where do you feel these sensations?
>
> What emotions are you currently experiencing as you integrate Reena's story into your body? Some emotions may include anger, sadness, confusion, anxiousness, and even numbness. When you feel these emotions and point them out to yourself, do the sensations in your body change, increasing, decreasing, or even moving to different parts of your body? Please feel free to record this information in your journal.
>
> For some of you this pause may seem impossible, because it is easier to move on to the next step versus truly feeling what comes up for you after reading such a traumatic experience. For others, the pause may seem like a relief, finally a time to feel with permission instead of hiding your emotion behind a wall of resilience and fight energy. In this space, learning how to pause is the foundation of moving this work from logical to somatic.

Why Did It Happen?

This story is familiar for many Black people who have lost a member of their family during the process of childbirth. We have seen *what* happened. Now let's look closely at the *why*.

Identity

The first place to look is at the identities of the characters within this story. Reena and her mother, Hilary, were both Black cis women. Both of them were college educated and middle class, from a suburb of Atlanta. Reena was born in the 1980s, while her mother was born in the '60s. Jarrod was a Black cis male born in the '80s. He was from Atlanta and did not have a college education. Samantha was a non-BIPOC cis woman originally from Massachusetts and had been a labor and delivery nurse for about ten years. Dr. Smith was a non-BIPOC cis man originally from Virginia, and he had been an ob-gyn for about twenty years. Knowing these identities, what imbalances of power and privilege present themselves?

The first thing you may notice is that Reena, Hilary, and Jarrod were Black, while their care providers were both non-BIPOC. This is not inherently a disadvantageous thing, but racial differences can bring up the possibilities of explicit and implicit bias, as well as an inability to understand cultural differences at play. One study, which examined 1.8 million hospital births in Florida between 1992 and 2015, found that Black infants cared for by Black doctors were *one-third less likely to die* than Black infants cared for by white doctors.[*] This outcome supports the importance of racially concordant care, which must be emphasized in a medical education system that currently rarely educates future physicians on racism and racial bias and their long-term effects on BIPOC folks seeking care. Racially concordant care is particularly hard to find in obstetrics, as ob-gyns have a shockingly low proportion of underrepresented minorities "(combined, 18.4%), especially black (11.1%) and Hispanic (6.7%)."[†]

---

[*] Brad N Greenwood et al., "Physician-Patient Racial Concordance and Disparities in Birthing Mortality for Newborns," *Proceedings of the National Academies of Sciences of the United States of America* 117, no. 35 (2020): 21194–21200, doi: 10.1073/pnas.1913405117.

[†] William F. Rayburn, "Racial and Ethnic Differences Between Obstetrician-Gynecologists and Other Adult Medical Specialists," *Obstetrics and Gynecology* 127, no 1. (2016): 148–152, doi: 10.1097/AOG.0000000000001184.

Power

This problem was further exacerbated by the power dynamics present in Reena's case. In Western medicine, doctors and nurses are the authority over the patient's body. Patients generally assume doctors and nurses automatically have this authority, given their care providers' extensive training and knowledge of the human body. So in this scenario, the doctor and the nurse inherently hold a lot of power in the room.

This power divide is even greater between white care providers and Black patients due to the historical abuse of Black bodies in Western medical history. Reena and Hilary entered this hospital room carrying with them the generational trauma of abuse and violence, even before anything happened to them. While Reena fully expected to receive proper care, she knew the history of white men and Black female bodies. It is impossible not to feel that history in every interaction, particularly one as vulnerable as birth. And of course, in our current medical system, physicians are not taught how to mitigate this trauma and power dynamic, and often don't even understand that it exists. "The Liaison Committee on Medical Education, the official accrediting body for medical schools in the U.S. and Canada, said faculty must teach students to recognize bias 'in themselves, in others, and in the health care delivery process.' But the LCME does not explicitly require accredited institutions to teach about systemic racism in medicine"[*]—so how can they actually achieve this?

It's also important to acknowledge that there are always power dynamics within families as well. If we don't allow ourselves to become aware and accept them, that can lead to unconscious harm. In this situation, there were a few dynamics at play: Hilary held parental power over Reena, as that had always been their dynamic, and Reena

---

[*] Elizabeth Lawrence, "What Doctors Aren't Always Taught: How to Spot Racism in Health Care," *KHN*, November 17, 2020, https://khn.org/news/racism-in-health-care-what-medical-schools-teach/.

was highly aware of Hilary feeling disrespected if Reena made any attempt to assert herself within their mother-daughter relationship. Hilary felt completely justified in sharing about her own traumatic birth and voicing her opinions on Reena's—even if this was not what Reena needed from her mother in this moment. Cis men like Jarrod too often feel unimportant and confused with all that is going on in an OB-GYN office, and they tend to check out or silently suffer while sometimes unknowingly leaving their partners unsupported and assuming their partner feels more knowledgeable about the experience, which isn't always true. Reena and Hilary, on the other hand, were more familiar in some ways with the hospital space; they knew the jargon of birth, and likely assumed not only that did Jarrod not know but also that he didn't *want* to know, which may or may not have been true.

On top of that, there was a layer of higher education. Reena and Hilary were able to navigate spaces differently because they attended college but Jarrod did not. When a BIPOC person has a bachelor's degree, it is common for that individual to become more skilled in navigating non-BIPOC people and people with more money due to it becoming somewhat of a survival skill in a higher education atmosphere. Jarrod's experience did not give him the tools to talk to medical staff in a confident way that would cause them to listen. He couldn't code-switch in the way that Reena and Hilary could.

Communication and Listening

Did you notice how Dr. Smith did not ask for consent before giving Reena a vaginal exam? How about when Reena and Jarrod both voiced concern over her headache and were dismissed? Or how Samantha noticed her blood pressure was a little high but told Reena she was just fine? Or how about Reena's mother, Hilary, who got swept into her memories of her own birth experience, which prevented her from being totally present for Reena and her needs?

I'm hoping at the very least you noticed that this death was 100 percent preventable and occurred due to lack of communication and awareness of the power dynamics at work within the room. In addition, each individual's trauma responses played a huge role in the outcome of this birth, and Reena is now another statistic of the Black perinatal mortality crisis.

The Trauma Perspective

It is very easy to place blame within specific situations and move quickly toward seeking "solutions" for next time that never end up working. We often do this in different areas in our lives beyond birth, such as when having a disagreement with our spouse, having difficulties with coworkers at our place of employment, or dealing with rifts in our families that seem to continue from generation to generation, never being processed or truly solved. A better way to approach these scenarios in order to effect real change moving forward is to reframe each individual experience from a trauma perspective. This is the only way we will find lasting solutions that will end the Black perinatal mortality crisis, as well as the additional ongoing traumas.

Reena

Prior to going into labor, Reena had planned for a vaginal birth without interventions. She chose this goal *because* of the perinatal statistics for Black birthing people. She could not financially afford a home birth, so although being in a hospital wasn't ideal, she had no other choice. When her birth plan went awry, Reena went into a state of freeze. Her fear of becoming another statistic combined with the lack of sensation from the waist down caused by the epidural led her to feel disconnected from her body and her mind. Being in freeze left her unable to be very responsive, such as when Dr. Smith gave her a vaginal exam without waiting for Reena to give him a clear yes or no. Reena knew about her mother's trauma and, out of concern for her, couldn't express her own needs or boundaries, or ask for the support she needed. Reena's headache did begin to take her out of freeze, but when her pain was dismissed, she fell further into her freeze response. As her headache got worse and she was given news of being scheduled for a C-section, Reena felt less and less present until her mind went blank. All she could hear around her was a jumble of voices until everything faded to black.

Jarrod

As a Black cis man from the city of Atlanta, Jarrod had been stereo-typed his whole life. He often experienced encounters where he was assumed, without reason, to be violent. Although Jarrod was very excited about meeting his son, he entered the situation carrying fear that he would be either ignored by Reena's care providers, dismissed as someone who wasn't knowledgeable enough to have an opinion, or even removed from the birthing room.

Through the years, Jarrod's own mother had experienced health emergencies that required her to be hospitalized. During a couple of these emergency hospital visits, after patiently waiting for assistance, Jarrod had urgently requested care for his mother, only to be removed from the premises by security guards for being "aggressive" and posing a threat to the staff. He quickly learned that voicing his opinion and demanding appropriate and urgent care in hospital spaces—while at the same time looking the way he did, with his Black skin—usually resulted in him being removed from the side of his loved one who needed him. During the interactions with Dr. Smith, Jarrod found himself wanting to say and do more, but his trauma around being seen as an Angry Black Man kept him in a state of freeze as well. Jarrod wanted a better expla-nation of the need for a cesarean section, and he wanted to demand more care for Reena when she voiced having a headache. But given his history, all he could do was nod his head, agree, and try to keep Hilary in a calm state. He was in freeze and operating at a very minimal level. He knew something felt off, but he didn't feel he could risk a conflict that could potentially have him removed from Reena's side.

In a study published in May 2022 in the *Journal of General Internal Medicine*, Black patients at Brigham and Women's Hospital in Boston experienced higher rates of security emergency responses compared with white patients.* A study that was done in 2018 discovered that patients in the hospital who were Black and had visitors had higher rates of security calls than white patients who had visitors.† These statistics indicate that the threat Jarrod felt was valid based not only on his life experience as a Black person but also on statistics that show the increase of police presence for Black families in hospital care.

This is the thing that haunts me now, I think about what if I had raised my voice, what if I had slammed on the counter, what if I had grabbed a doctor by his collar? But the entire time I was thinking, I've got to stay calm because if I raise my voice as an African American male I become seen as a threat. I think about, well, what if I had been kicked out and then the same result ensued? I would never be able to live with myself and who would be there fighting for my wife, right? So there's all these layers that as an African American man we don't even have the latitude or the autonomy to express

---

* Yannis K. Valtis et al., "Race and Ethnicity and the Utilization of Security Responses in a Hospital Setting," *Journal of General Internal Medicine* (2022), https://doi.org/10.1007/s11606-022-07525-1.

† Jessica Bartlett, "Internal Analysis Shows Black Patients at Brigham Faced More Security Calls," *The Boston Globe*, May 23 2022, https://www.bostonglobe.com/2022/05/23/metro/black-patients-brigham-womens-are-nearly-twice-likely-have-security-called-them-white-patients/.

ourselves when it is the most critical situation. And the people
that depend on us, you know, I didn't feel like I had the ability
to fight for my wife like I really felt I should have.

—Charles Johnson, founder of 4Kira4Moms and husband
    of Kira Johnson, a Black mother who died during
    childbirth of preventable causes*

Hilary

Since the announcement of Reena's pregnancy, Hilary was excited
but apprehensive. She was more than ready to be a grandmother
but fearful of the experience Reena might have during her labor.
She wanted to have faith that Reena would be treated properly and
not experience a racist health care team in the way she did. But as
Reena got closer to her due date, Hilary began to have flashbacks
and nightmares about her own birth experience. She chose not to tell
Reena about these because she didn't want to scare or upset Reena.
She promised her daughter that she would be present throughout
her entire labor.

When the time came for Hilary to attend Reena's birth, she was
feeling tense, frustrated, and anxious. Upon seeing that Reena's care
team consisted entirely of non-BIPOC people, Hilary was immediately triggered, and began to unknowingly compare every aspect of
Reena's experience with her own experience years before. When Dr.
Smith suggested a C-section, Hilary had a visceral reaction against
it, though Reena and Jarrod initially were more open to it. Hilary
got even more frustrated when Jarrod insinuated that she needed to
calm down, especially since, in her opinion, he wasn't doing enough
to advocate for Reena. Hilary did go outside to try to calm down, but

---

* Charles Johnson, "Black Mothers Matter: Racism and Childbirth in America," BBM
  Panel, *Hollywood Health and Society*, May 21, 2019, audio, 37:34, https://youtu.be
  /DVi46ErwY00.

the moments away from her daughter made her even more anxious, putting her even further into fight mode and triggering her to share about her own traumatic birth experience at the worst possible time.

Nurse Samantha

Samantha loved being a labor and delivery nurse and had always felt blessed to love a job that also helped her care for her own four children so well. She had experienced homelessness when she was younger; becoming a nurse changed the course of her life and allowed her to create a good life for her children.

Over her years of experience, she had been present for hundreds of births. Her philosophy, as a mom and birth worker, was to trust the birthing person and try to assist them in having the birth experience they were hoping for. Knowing that Reena was a first-time mom, Samantha was not alarmed by the length of her labor. She was also heavily aware of the Black perinatal mortality rates in the United States, so she was aligned with Reena's goal of having a vaginal birth. She felt she was doing all she could for Reena while at the same time completing the continuous charting that had to be done throughout the process. Samantha often wished she could do less charting so she could be more present for her patients. Dr. Smith was famous among the nurses for his impatience, so Samantha was consistently aware of her duty to keep him happy. When Samantha learned of Reena's headache and noticed that her blood pressure was a little higher than it should be, she brushed it off as a normal response to stress and then went back to charting and giving an update to Dr. Smith. When Dr. Smith initially told Samantha to schedule the C-section, she immediately went into a fight response. She felt tightness in her chest and anger in her heart, especially after hearing Reena say that she felt like a failure. Samantha felt protective of Reena and was frustrated when Dr. Smith opted for surgery when Reena was progressing. Feeling it was her duty on Reena's behalf, she took a risk of violating protocol and told Dr. Smith her opinion. But he didn't move his eyes from the computer screen, which made her feel belittled and dismissed. When Dr. Smith responded by enforcing his authority, Samantha worried for her job and quickly shifted into a fawn response. She told him that yes, of course his decision was the right one, even though that's not at all what she believed. She didn't want to cause any long-term issues between her and Dr. Smith since they worked together often. She needed this job for her and her family's survival. What other choice did she have? All these feelings further distracted her from the issue of Reena's headache instead of creating a commonality of discomfort between herself and Reena that could have increased her empathy and motivated her to pay closer attention to Reena's symptoms.

Dr. Smith

Dr. Smith had been an ob-gyn for twenty years leading up to his interaction with Reena. He got his education from a program that did not discuss the violent history of gynecology, racial disparities in health care, or the Black perinatal mortality crisis. As a non-BIPOC male physician, Dr. Smith had always been the authority in his position and expected nothing different in this scenario.

While he was treating Reena, he focused on following hospital procedures, one of which was scheduling a C-section if a labor goes over thirty-six hours. Earlier in his career, he once went against this policy, thinking a client would be fine even though she had been in labor for forty-eight hours. Unfortunately this patient died unexpectedly from a pregnancy complication. Her death caused him to go into a deep depression, and he'd never forgotten the experience. Since then, he has followed hospital policies without question. To his understanding, hospital policies were created to ensure that patients have the best possible outcome while under his care.

When Hilary questioned his decision-making by asking for his reasoning for the C-section, he automatically went into fight response. Feeling threatened, he tersely explained his answer and demonstrated his authority. He had been taught that his job was to diagnose and to treat—end of story. His lack of education around racism and Black perinatal mortality rates left him blind to the valid fears that Reena and her family were experiencing, so he was unable to be sensitive to their concerns. His training had taught him that being emotionally connected to a patient would only harm his ability to see the situation clearly. He believed he was doing his job by quickly coming in to complete his task and exit just as quickly, thereby avoiding any emotional reactions and leaving the support role to Nurse Samantha.

After Reena's death, Dr. Smith questioned if he should have done anything differently, but he quickly stopped that thought, reminding himself that in his profession death sometimes happens. When he confronted the family with the news of Reena's death, Dr. Smith used the words he always uses. Their pain triggered flight response, and he felt his muscles tense and the strong urge to walk away. With his heart racing, he quickly left to check on his next patient, once again trying to leave emotion out of his work.

———————

You see now how diving deeper into the trauma experience of each person creates a layered understanding of the situation. I hope this story illustrates how *everyone* experiences traumas that influence the way they interact and react in the present. This truth is at the heart of reproductive justice. This truth is the path to collective liberation. I dare say it might be the answer to everything.

2

HISTORY OF RACE AND GYNECOLOGY

The truth is powerful and will prevail.

—Sojourner Truth, *Narrative of Sojourner Truth;*
A Bondwoman of Olden Time, Emancipated by the New York Legislature
in the Early Part of the Present Century; with a History of Her Labors and
Correspondence Drawn from Her "Book of Life"

I'M A FIRM BELIEVER in understanding history before moving forward. Learning the history of race and gynecology will allow us to understand the roots of present-day disparities and complications while also informing us on what has been tried to improve the health and lives of Black families, successful or not. I also recognize that much of the history that you will be reading about will have a great chance of making you feel uncomfortable, angry, and many other negative emotions, so before we dive into this history, I would like you to take a moment to create a plan for that discomfort. Remember, this work isn't about rushing through the content just to say you recall all the historical details, it's about consuming the information both intellectually and somatically in order to build a whole-body experience of knowledge.

Let's start first with creating an environment that cares for you. That may look like a fuzzy blanket, making sure your bottle of water is full, emptying your bladder, turning on a specific type of music or lighting a candle. Next, I want you to practice a couple of the following suggestions while reading through this chapter.

If you begin to feel discomfort in any of your body while reading, pause and take deep breaths, breathing into the discomfort and not away from it. If breathing does not seem to decrease the sensations, I welcome you to move your body to your ability. That may look like a full body shake, tapping your foot, rolling your neck, or whatever feels right to you in the moment. Don't overthink it. Just let it happen.

If needed, take a break and make a plan to return to this book. This is especially important for BIPOC folks because this is our history, these are our bodies and our current lived experiences. We are often faced with having to endure pain without pause, even in educational spaces. Pause as much as you like and need to. There is space for you and your well-being here.

Lastly, the language available to us in this chapter will unfortunately be very gendered to maintain the context of the history I will share. Gender nonconforming and transgender people very much existed and made great impact during these historical times but were not respected or centered in the ways they should have been.

This chapter isn't supposed to be easy to read. Part of the reason why we are in the space we are right now is because of the whitewashing, simplifying, and erasure of Black history. Remember, Black history is AMERICAN history.

The Beginning

In the year 1619, the first few ships carrying about thirty enslaved Africans each arrived in what is now known as Fort Monroe in Hampton, Virginia.* These events marked the beginning of Black bodies being treated as property: less than human and only valuable—only making a contribution—when performing a task connected to the increased power, money, and knowledge of non-BIPOC people.

What does that actually mean? *Contribution* implies a voluntary act. There was nothing voluntary here. Black women were forced every step of the way—conceiving their children through rape, being forced to carry those children of rape through to term, and then being unable to feed those children because their breast milk was being co-opted by the non-BIPOC children of their rapists.

That was the baseline experience of a Black enslaved woman.

Black birthing people nowadays have access to better health care than their enslaved ancestors, though let's remember it is by no means as high quality as a non-BIPOC birthing person's health care. But the uncomfortable truth is that much of modern reproductive health care

---

* Beth Austin, "1619: Virginia's First Africans," Hampton History Museum: Make History with Us, December 31, 2019, 3, https://hampton.gov/DocumentCenter/View/24075/1619 -Virginias-First-Africans?bidId=.

was developed through experimentation on the bodies of enslaved Black women.

So is that contribution? Or is that torture?

Is it a contribution to suffer through an unnecessary C-section? Is it a contribution to be forced to hold down one of your friends, someone you are in community with, while she is operated on again and again, without anesthetic?

None of this is an exaggeration.

J. Marion Sims, also known as the Father of Gynecology, has been praised for inventing the speculum, the Sims position, and the vesicovaginal fistula surgery in the time when reproductive health was not seen as a notable focus. In fact, it was seen as inappropriate to focus on "women's issues" at that time.* The people who have not been credited nearly enough for these inventions are the enslaved Black women whose bodies were used to bring these inventions to life.

Sims started his path into gynecological care when a patient fell off a horse, which resulted in ongoing pelvic and back pain. During his examination of the client, he realized the client was suffering from a vesicovaginal fistula. A vesicovaginal fistula is an abnormal infected tract extending between the bladder and vagina that causes the constant and involuntary release of urine. It can be the consequence of a vaginal or bladder injury and can have major physical and emotional effects on the affected person. There was no known cure for this ailment, and this incident set Sims forward on the path to doing experimental surgeries on enslaved Black women who suffered from this injury.†

Over the four years it took Sims to become "successful" with inventing the vesicovaginal fistula repair surgery, he performed

---

* Jeffrey S. Sartin, "J. Marion Sims, the Father of Gynecology: Hero or Villain?," *Southern Medical Journal* 97, no. 5 (2004): 500–505, doi: 10.1097/00007611-200405000-00017.

† John Spurlock, "Vesicovaginal Fistula," *Medscape*, November 11, 2021, https://emedicine.medscape.com/article/267943-overview.

surgeries on many enslaved Black women. Three of the most well-known and documented women are Lucy, Betsy, and Anarcha, who worked on three different plantations in Montgomery, Alabama. Slaves with this injury were kept separate from the rest of the slaves because it made them worthless since they were unable to produce work efficiently or reproduce more children for their slaveholder's plantation. Enslavers were frustrated by losing "manpower" and sought a solution by leasing Lucy, Betsy, and Anarcha to J. Marion Sims with the hopes that he would "fix" them and business could continue to run smoothly. Remember, slaves were either a commodity or collateral, which means there was no time for injury or anything that slowed down their ability to involuntarily give their body, mind, and spirit to the advancement of non-BIPOC people.

Lucy was the first enslaved Black woman Sims operated on. Lucy, unfortunately, had a vesicovaginal fistula as a result of giving birth a few months previously. With permission from Lucy's slaveholders, Sims performed an unsuccessful and agonizing hour-long surgery. He made Lucy take off all her clothing and get on all fours with her head balanced on her elbows while she screamed in pain and he performed the surgery with an audience of other doctors present. (It is important to note that at this time, in 1845, anesthesia was not available. It was also widely believed Black people didn't feel the pain as non-BIPOC people did, and there were of course non-BIPOC people who did not care about Black people and their pain. In 1846 anesthesia became available, but Sims chose not to use this option throughout these experimental surgeries.)

Lucy became very ill after this surgery due to Sims using a sponge to drain the urine away from the bladder, which resulted in blood poisoning. Sims and others believed that Lucy would die. She "recovered" from the surgery a couple of months later but did not see any improvements in her fistula. The operation was unsuccessful.

The torture of enslaved Black women continued with Betsy. Betsy experienced the same agonizing surgery, but Sims did not use a sponge to drain the urine away from her bladder. Fortunately, she did not experience any major infections, but her injury did not improve. Another failed surgery for Sims.

Anarcha, a seventeen-year-old enslaved woman who experienced a traumatic birth that resulted in a vesicovaginal fistula, is undoubtedly the most well-known enslaved woman Sims operated on. She, of course, is not known for any of her qualities but for the number of surgeries Sims performed on her—twenty-nine agonizing and anesthesia-free failures, to be exact. Complete torture that still resulted in no relief from her injury.

After Anarcha's failed surgeries, many of Sims's colleagues and assistants decided to disconnect from the doctor because he was now deemed a failure. I would personally like to think that his colleagues also realized how inhumane Sims's practices were and walked away because of their morals, but that has yet to be determined.

Without any success in these initial surgeries, Sims was left without a team of doctors and assistants to help him continue these experiments. He was also now the enslaver of Lucy, Betsy, and Anarcha because their original enslavers did not want the women to return with their injuries still keeping them from work. Sims decided to keep these three women as his slaves, and he even trained them to be assistants, which meant they would hold each other and other enslaved women down during these experimental and extremely painful surgeries. Finally, in the summer of 1849, Sims performed Anarcha's thirtieth surgery, and it was a success. From there, Sims publicized his surgery method and returned Lucy, Betsy, and Anarcha to their original slaveholders before moving to the North.*

---

* "Life Story: Anarcha, Betsy, and Lucy: The Mothers of Modern Gynecology," *Women and the American Story*, https://wams.nyhistory.org/a-nation-divided/antebellum/anarcha-betsy-lucy/#resource.

Before we continue, I would like to mention that even with the documented stories of Lucy, Betsy, and Anarcha, there are supporters of J. Marion Sims. These supporters, such as L. L. Wall, professor of anthropology at Washington University, believe that the experiments that Sims performed were voluntary and desired by the enslaved women who suffered from vesicovaginal fistulas. In his article "The Obstetric Vesicovaginal Fistula in the Developing World," Wall argues,

> It is true that under Southern law, slaves were the property of others and Sims could not have legally operated on them without the consent of their owners; however, this cannot be taken as a priori proof that these slaves were unwilling patients. As a matter of surgical practicality, considering the delicate and tedious requirements of performing surgery inside the vagina and the exceedingly difficult circumstances of exposure and inadequate lighting under which he was forced to operate, Sims could not have carried out these operations successfully without the cooperation of the women involved. Even the slightest movement, much less the active resistance of these patients, would have rendered it impossible for him to have completed his operative procedures.*

Can consent truly be given when under the rule of another that has the power to negatively affect, even end, your life and the lives of community members without consequence? Hold on to this question as we move along. It will be an important one that we will ask again and again.

* L. Lewis Wall, "The Medical Ethics of Dr. J. Marion Sims: A Fresh Look at the Historical Record," *Journal of Medical Ethics* 32, no. 6 (2006): 346–350, https://doi.org/10.1136/jme.2005.012559.

Somatic Practice: Building Capacity for Discomfort

As I mentioned at the beginning of this chapter, the history of gynecology and its direct connection to the centuries-long abuse and violation of Black bodies will bring up many feelings of discomfort. In American culture, there is traditionally an avoidance of discomfort. We, and I include myself, tend to push that discomfort to the side hoping to find relief, in sometimes not-so-healthy ways. I have learned that fully feeling discomfort is one of the keys to being liberated. When we allow our feelings to direct our actions, we are not acting from a place of liberation, so I welcome you to move through the feelings of discomfort you are experiencing right now after reading through the treacherous experiences of Lucy, Betsy, and Anarcha.

According to Conscious Leadership Group, "a cognitive/emotive loop is a repeating pattern where thoughts and beliefs produce feelings that fuel our rightness about our stories, that then further intensify our feelings, and on and on. They burn energy and get in the way of progress. They're one way we as humans get stuck."* In this next exercise, we are aiming to move through this stuckness, and it is important for you to know it takes ninety seconds to identify an emotion and allow it to dissipate while you simply notice it. This is not to say that after ninety seconds you will experience fits of joy, but being able to move through these ninety seconds will allow you to name your emotion and gain more control over yourself and what you want to do with that emotion, allowing you to move beyond stuckness, discomfort, righteousness—and into positive action.

---

* Jim Dethmer, "The Cognitive Emotive Loop: What It Is, Why It Keeps You Stuck, and How to Break Free," Conscious Leadership Group, March 21, 2018, https://conscious.is/blogs/the-cognitive-emotive-loop-what-it-is-why-it-keeps-you-stuck-and-how-to-break-free.

Riding the Emotional Wave Meditation

1. When you notice you are having a feeling of discomfort, pause and take notice of what physical sensations you are feeling in your body. Name these sensations to yourself (i.e., tightness in your chest, tingly hands and feet, tension in your upper back).
2. After naming the physical sensations to yourself, name the feeling connected to those sensations. You can use the simple phrase "I am feeling [insert emotion]." It is also OK to say something such as "I am not sure what I am feeling, but I am still acknowledging my general feeling of discomfort."
3. After naming the feeling, allow the feeling to come and go without judgment. What that means is not passing judgment on yourself for having a "wrong" or "big" feeling, and instead giving yourself permission to feel with the goal of regaining or maintaining your personal sense of groundedness.
4. If you would like, journal your additional thoughts or feelings or take part in a coping mechanism that is positive for you and provides additional comfort.

Use this exercise as you continue moving through this book, understanding that the path to liberation isn't ignoring your feelings and overriding them with action. Instead, it is feeling your feelings, naming them, and learning how to operate with them as a part of your overall being.

Sims is by no means the only doctor to experiment on enslaved women's bodies in this way: "A slaveholding surgeon, François Marie Prevost, pioneered cesarean section surgeries on American enslaved women's bodies through repeated experimentation."* There are also ongoing

---

* Deirdre Cooper Owens and Sharla M. Fett, "Black Maternal and Infant Health: Historical Legacies of Slavery," *American Journal of Public Health* 109, no. 10 (2019), 1343, doi: 10.2105/AJPH.2019.305243.

findings of doctors experimenting with amputations and other surgeries without anesthesia before these surgeries became part of standard practice. This unfortunately was a normal occurrence at the time, and how many slaves were affected by these experiments is yet to be fully known.

Black Family During Enslavement

I would be remiss if I wrote this book without mentioning the life of enslaved Black families and the trauma that came from these experiences. During the almost 250 years of enslavement, Black families were tasked with the challenge of creating and maintaining families, sometimes involuntarily and sometimes with the hopes of providing a level of normalcy and closeness while under bondage.

Slaveholders depended on enslaved women to continue reproducing children so they could continue running their businesses and maintain their livelihoods. At the time, marriage was not legal for enslaved Black adults, but that did not keep slaveholders from forcing and allowing involuntary and voluntary relationships between enslaved women and men. Some enslaved adults did not have the ability to pick who they were forced into a "marriage" with, and refusal of these arrangements would result in many consequences, such as being sold to another owner and even death. In these arranged marriages, slaves would have to deal with forcing themselves to both mentally and physically engage with each other, even if they were uninterested or had a different person who they were voluntarily in relationship with.*

Some slaveholders allowed enslaved people to choose the person they would "marry" and create their own family with. To many slaves this seemed like a gift, but this gift still remained tied to bondage and

---

* Dorothy Roberts, *Killing the Black Body: Race Reproduction and the Meaning of Liberty* (New York: Vintage Books, 1997), 28.

the direct benefit of non-BIPOC people. Some slaveholders believed that allowing enslaved people to pick and choose their own family would result in happier slaves and would reduce the chance of there being any issues, such as disobedience or revolts. This is partially true. Many slaves found solace in being able to build families and share those moments we all want to experience, like being able to spend time with their partners and children, though they were still limited by the bondage that defined their lives.

There were also difficulties and challenges that chosen enslaved Black families dealt with. One major issue was the separation of families, a constant threat that always lingered in the air. It was not unusual for a family member to be sold to another slaveholder in exchange for goods and services, debt repayment, etc. For example, a father would be sold to another slaveholder and would be tasked with finding time to walk miles to see his children or, at other times, would never see his children again. For some slaveholders, there were benefits to keeping families separated, such as being able to manipulate a slave to do anything at the chance of being able to see their family members or simply keeping the spirit of a slave broken because the one thing that gave them hope no longer existed.

In the 1850s many Black individuals had to make a hard decision—remain free or become "voluntarily" reenslaved for their families. At the time, many former slaves had escaped to the North for their freedom, but their family members were still enslaved in the South; this was known as a *mixed status* family. In the antebellum South, "free" former slaves were targeted by an ongoing battle with laws that legally required them to choose either to be reenslaved or to leave their home state, which also meant leaving their enslaved family members behind. As you can tell, freedom was really an illusion at this point and a way for non-BIPOC people to manipulate free former slaves back into slavery voluntarily. Some former slaves did leave the state, never to see their families again, and some left the state and eventually returned to voluntarily become enslaved again because they could not live their lives without their families.

We must also keep in mind that through these different choices and shifts that Black families had to make and see through, there was also the abuse and rape of Black enslaved women. Black women being forced to have sexual relationships with their slaveholders. Some having children by their slaveholders while being in their voluntary or involuntary families. Black women being forced to prioritize feeding their milk to slaveholders' children and to care for them several hours a day while hoping their children were being taken care of by other slaves. Black fathers and community members seeing each other be brutalized and not being able to do much about it. Black children being made to work as early as they could walk and talk. Black children being physically, mentally, and emotionally abused by their slaveholders. Constant and endless traumas being experienced and absorbed while still trying to maintain the richness and importance of family.

In 1815 Henry Brown was born enslaved in Louisa County, Virginia. He was sent to work in a tobacco factory at the age of fifteen where he eventually met his wife, Nancy. Nancy was also enslaved and lived on a plantation adjacent to Henry's. Henry and Nancy had several children, and unfortunately, while Nancy was pregnant with their fourth child, Henry and Nancy received the news that Nancy and their children had been sold to a North Carolina plantation. Henry had no say in the matter and had to witness his wife and children leaving, most likely never to be seen by him again. This experience infuriated him and further emphasized how helpless he was to save them as well as how much the slave masters did not care about him or his family. Henry decided the only way he could survive this treacherous life was to escape. Henry created a plan of escape and recruited a fellow church member, James Caesar Anthony Smith, to assist him with his plan. The plan was for Henry to get himself shipped in a box from Richmond, Virginia, to Philadelphia, Pennsylvania, where he could be free. James knew a white sympathizer, Samuel Alexander Smith, who decided to assist with the plan in exchange for profit to fund him in his gambling habit. Samuel then contacted a non-BIPOC abolitionist and experienced member of the Philadelphia Anti-Slavery Society, James Miller McKim. Henry was sent to Richmond in a wooden box—3' long by 2'8" deep by 2' wide—labeled DRY GOODS by Adams Express Company on March 23, 1849. The box had a hole for air flow and was lined with a coarse woolen cloth and contained Henry, some water, and a few biscuits. The journey to Philadelphia took twenty-seven hours and included modes of transportation such as railroads, steamboats, and ferries. Henry later expressed the physical chaos of the box being tossed around violently and also the mental anguish of the fear of being caught and punished. Through it all, he completed his box journey and became a free man. He then became known as Henry "Box" Brown.*

We could never FULLY feel all the feelings enslaved and "free" Black individuals and families felt at this time, but for a moment, I want you to imagine the weight of these experiences and notice what sensations take place in your body. Imagine being forced into arranged marriages that literally mandated reproduction for the financial stability and gain of non-BIPOC people. Imagine being able to choose your family and have those moments of closeness, happiness, and affection, only for that to be overshadowed by the fact that your life isn't really your own and the well-being of your family depended on how efficient and valuable your slave owner thought you to be. Imagine being pregnant and not knowing if the father of your child is your husband that you love and cherish or the slaveholder that you hate

---

* Bryan Walls, "Freedom Marker: Courage and Creativity," *Underground Railroad: The William Still Story*, PBS, accessed June 15, 2022, https://www.pbs.org/black-culture/shows /list/underground-railroad/stories-freedom/henry-box-brown/.

but can't avoid. Imagine raising children only to wonder when their bodies will become a commodity and knowing neither you nor they have any control over their bodies or their lives. Imagine having to hold on to the fear that your family can be separated at any moment without any warning, for any reason. Imagine being a Black father and being sold off to another slaveholder and wondering if you will ever have the ability to see your family again. Imagine being the mother to those children and having to explain why they will never see their father again. Imagine going through hell to become free, thinking your life is about to begin again, just to be told you now have to choose between your freedom and your family.

This was the reality of Black people for centuries.

Post-Slavery

African women with generational knowledge about reproductive health and childbirth were among the slaves transported to North America. During the centuries of slavery, these women, also known as midwives, continued to pass down the knowledge and skills of midwifery. These African enslaved women had the responsibility of caring for not only the enslaved community but also the community of non-BIPOC slaveholders. These women also assisted with lactation, birth complications, and general care, and they were valued in their enslaved community.

When slavery ended, these women became known as Granny midwives. Although slavery was outlawed, Black people were still facing racism, discrimination, abuse, denial of care, and more. Granny midwives became the matriarchs in their communities, especially in southern and rural Black communities. At the same time that Granny midwives were continuing their work in the 1800s, health care was becoming more industrialized. This meant that physicians were now beginning to be more present and take a bigger stake in gynecology and obstetrics, especially with white upper- and middle-class patients' experience of childbirth. In the early 1900s, high perinatal mortality and infant mortality rates began to plague the medical-industrial complex, and Granny midwives were blamed. Although the research at the time showed a lesser chance of mortality during births attended by midwives, the blame was still put on midwives instead of the incompetence of poorly trained physicians who did not have enough knowledge or practice to guarantee safety to birthing people. This falsified information and stigma led to the public campaign against the practice of midwifery in the United States.* While midwives were being ousted and punished unfairly in the United States, places like Britain were creating and formalizing the practice of nurse midwifery in order to maintain low perinatal and infant mortality in line with what current research had shown.

In the United States, the reality was babies were always going to be born and there was lots of money in being able to industrialize and medicalize the childbirth process, especially if birth was moved from the home to the hospital. This realization along with the public campaign against midwives began to push Granny midwives out of the birthing space more and more by creating legislation in states that outlawed the practice of lay midwives.

The traditional practices of Granny midwives typically reflect those of a lay midwife, an apprentice who learns from a practicing midwife, gaining hands-on knowledge rather than receiving credentials from a formal midwifery school. These laws had a major impact on Granny midwives, who in the 1940s were attending up to 70 percent of the births in their southeastern communities.† Only a few years later, Granny midwives ceased to exist, and Black birthing people now had to interact with the medical-industrial complex to receive care. Black birthing people interacting with the medical-industrial complex often

---

* Margaret Charles Smith and Linda Janet Holmes, *Listen to Me Good: The Story of an Alabama Midwife* (Columbus, OH: Ohio State University Press, 1996), 64.

† Smith and Holmes, *Listen to Me Good*, 64.

had to deal with abuse of all kinds, being denied care and facing discrimination and racism. So although Granny midwives had to legally stop practicing, many continued practicing illegally with the risk of punishment because their communities needed them.*

Onnie Lee Logan was born into a lineage of midwives. Her mother was a midwife, and her grandmother, who was enslaved, was also a midwife. Onnie Lee Logan became a passionate and well-known midwife in Alabama. Although she helped deliver most of the children in the Black areas of Mobile, Alabama, for over fifty years, she still had to maintain a domestic servant job with a local physician's family to support herself and her family. In 1949 she received her midwife permit in Mobile, Alabama; until that time permits weren't necessary to practice midwifery. She received her permit to practice faster than any other midwife because of her twenty years of experience. She was proud of that fact and often mentioned that two-thirds of her knowledge to pass the midwifery examinations progressed out of her own mind, and she contributed that intuitive knowing to God. In 1915 most states had begun to outlaw lay midwives due to the pressure of the medical system believing physicians needed to be the only medical provider for birthing people, regardless of the positive statistics attributed to midwifery care. In 1976 Alabama outlawed lay midwives, but Onnie Lee Logan, one of the last midwives in the country, was able to practice until 1984. She, like many Black midwives at the time, did not believe in the outlawing of midwives and understood the importance of their work continuing with or without permission for the literal survival of their communities. Many midwives of this period went rogue and continued to practice underground, and many dealt with the consequences of being caught, understanding that this was the necessary work of a Black midwife in America.† As Onnie Lee Logain defiantly said:

---

* Smith and Holmes, *Listen to Me Good*, 67.

† Onnie Lee Logan and Katherine Clark, *Motherwit: An Alabama Midwife's Story* (Belmont, CA: Untreed Reads Publishing, 2014); Steven J. Niven, "Motherwit: Onnie Lee Logan's

They're not going to stop me from doing the gift that God give me to do. I don't be going there on no license. I be going there as a friend to help that husband deliver his baby.*

As the ousting and outlawing of Granny midwives continued, the mainstream medical system created barriers to becoming a midwife. Schools of midwifery were established that did not allow Black people and other BIPOC communities to attend, and even if they did, the amount of emotional abuse would make sure they did not want to return. There were also barriers to receiving a legal midwifery education such as the cost to attend school, the accessibility of school locations, and the levels of reading and writing required to get through the school process. There was no room for Black midwives to thrive and continue the service they had provided to their communities for centuries, through enslavement and post-enslavement. The same knowledge they had brought to North America when they were forced into slavery was now being used to keep them away from their traditional practices and was also weakening the state of the Black community that would afterward have to depend on colonial systems to provide care during the intimate experience of childbirth.

Although Black people were free at this time and had begun to establish their own communities with service providers such as Granny midwives, the commodification of Black bodies persisted. When slavery ended, many Black birthing people could not receive care at any non-BIPOC institutions, even in life-or-death situations. However, when the ability to commodify Black people presented itself

---

4 Decades as a Midwife in Ala.," *The Root*, March 28, 2016, https://www.theroot.com /motherwit-onnie-lee-logan-s-4-decades-as-a-midwife-in-1790854770.

* Nina Renata Aron, "Meet the Unheralded Women Who Saved Mothers' Lives and Delivered Babies Before Modern Medicine," *Timeline*, January 11, 2018, https://timeline.com µ/granny-midwives-birthed-rural-babies-and-saved-lives-33f12601ba84.

in industrializing health care, medicalizing the childbirth experience and moving childbirth from mostly at home to mostly at the hospital, the value of Black bodies went up. Once again, Black bodies would be used for the financial gain of non-BIPOC people by commodifying their health through medical bills and supplies, creating a dependence on a medical system that in the past did not want them to be present or to utilize its services.

Obstetric Violence

Obstetric violence takes place any time a pregnant or laboring person experiences mistreatment or a mispractice of their rights. Any medical staff, including physicians and all types of midwives, can commit obstetric violence by perpetrating physical, sexual, or verbal abuse, bullying, coercion, humiliation, or assault. This can range from a hostile doula all the way to a forced medical procedure. None of it is more or less important or impactful—it all counts, and all can lead to a strong trauma response.

Take note that in the beginning of slavery, Black birthing people did not have any bodily autonomy and were forced to endure abuse of any kind, ranging from rape to using their bodies to feed the children of their enslavers. However, Black enslaved birthing people did have human rights, and those rights were not respected in any sense of the word. Human rights are universal rights we have because we exist as human beings—they are not granted by legal entities. Some of the most basic human rights include the rights to be free, to not be tortured, to not be enslaved, and to be safe—rights that were not acknowledged or respected under slavery. As time progressed and slavery became outlawed, Black communities depended on Granny midwives for many reasons: lower perinatal and infant mortality rates, culturally appropriate care, and safety. The commodification of Black bodies during the industrialization and medicalization of childbirth reintroduced a high level of obstetric violence into the lives of the Black community. I say "reintroduced" because no provider is exempt from knowingly or unknowingly committing obstetric violence, but we do know now that racially concordant care is helpful for decreasing infant mortality rates and increasing the overall experience of patients. Joy Cooper, an ob-gyn and founder of Culture Care,* shared that a 2017 study published in the *Journal of Racial and Ethnic Health Disparities* found that when the doctor and patient share the same racial identity there is overall better communication,† and a "2020 study in Florida found that Black infants were more likely to survive if they were cared for by a Black pediatrician," proving that racially concordant care could be one of many tools used to assist in the health and longevity of Black community members by creating spaces of safety and understanding.‡

Cristen Pascucci, the creator of Birth Monopoly (an organization focused on the awareness and elimination of obstetric violence around the globe), states that there are three forms of obstetric violence: normalization, degradation, and assault. Normalization can include trivializing pain, using coercion to influence a birthing person's choice, and presenting routine procedures with implied consent. Degradation can include bullying, intimidation, and ignoring questions, pleas, or requests by the birthing person. Assault can include legal coercion, forced procedures, and the use of physical force.** This list of obstetric

---

* Joy Cooper, "Racially-Concordant Care: Why It Matters if Your Provider Looks Like You," For Families (blog), Hi Cleo, February 1, 2021, https://hicleo.com/resource/racially-concordant-care-why-it-matters-if-your-provider-looks-like-you.

† Megan Johnson Shen, et al., "The Effects of Race and Racial Concordance on Patient-Physician Communication: A Systematic Review of the Literature," *Journal of Racial and Ethnic Health Disparities* 5, no. 1 (2018): 117–140, doi: 10.1007/s40615-017-0350-4.

‡ Cooper, "Racially-Concordant Care."

** Birth Monopoly, "Obstetric Violence," accessed June 15, 2022, https://birthmonopoly.com/obstetric-violence/.

violence is not at all exhaustive, but we can use these examples to reflect back on what we have learned within this chapter.

Historically Black bodies have been used illegally and forcibly to the advancement of non-BIPOC people. Black birthing people have had to silently suffer from obstetric violence and other forms of violence since their involuntary arrival in North America. Granny midwives stood in as pillars to our communities and as symbols of the freedom Black people had lost for 250 years. However, that symbol of freedom served as a threat to non-BIPOC people and the systems built to support the continuation of white supremacy, which led to the exile of Granny midwives and the increase of childbirth as a colonized, industrialized, and medicalized process. What once was an intimate experience involving the safety and love of the community was no longer. Black birthing people were forced into a system that was not built for them and didn't prioritize them but would continuously and ongoingly provide financial security and growth to systems built by and for non-BIPOC communities.

Before moving on to the next chapter, I suggest you take a minute to once again practice pausing, naming your emotions, and creating space for whatever it is you need at this moment—whether it be a break from this book, writing out your thoughts in a notebook, or some physical movement—before continuing. This book is not a race; it is a journey.

3

PRESENT-DAY PERSPECTIVE

THE RACIAL DIVIDE

Not everything that is faced can be changed; but nothing can be changed until it is faced.

—James Baldwin, "As Much Truth as One Can Bear"

L ET'S TOUCH ON these statistics again.
  Black birthing people are three to four times more likely to die from a pregnancy-related cause than white birthing people. The chance that Black infants will die in their first year of life is two to three times that for white infants. In places like Wisconsin, which has the worst record in the nation for Black infant mortality,* perinatal mortality for Black birthing people is five times higher than for white birthing people.[†]

Black birthing people are also less likely to bodyfeed compared with white and Hispanic birthing people. According to the CDC, "fewer non-Hispanic Black infants (75.5%) are ever breastfed compared with Asian infants (92.4%), non-Hispanic White infants (85.3%) and His-panic infants (85.0%)."[‡] I'll discuss further why this is a problem—and why it's not the fault of those parents who don't bodyfeed.

We can all agree that these statistics are disappointing and infu-riating, to say the least. However, a habit that I have seen coming from performative and well-meaning organizations, all types of birth workers, and people meaning to do good is plastering these statistics everywhere but not spending the time to figure out the why, the how, and what actions would change the direction of these statistics in a positive and long-lasting way.

It personally enrages me and retraumatizes me to see visual rep-resentation of members of BIPOC communities in medical spaces, social media, and those handy-dandy pamphlets only in reference to

---

* Dane County Health Council, "Dane County Health Council and Partners Announce Black Maternal and Child Health Alliance to Lead Local Birth Equity Efforts," *University of Wisconsin-Madison News*, September 18, 2020, https://news.wisc.edu/dane-county -health-council-and-partners-announce-historic-launch-of-the-black-maternal-and -child-health-alliance-to-lead-local-birth-equity-efforts/.

† Michael A Schellpfeffer et al., "A Review of Pregnancy-Related Maternal Mortality in Wisconsin, 2006–2010," *Wisconsin Medical Journal* 114, no. 5 (2015): 202–207.

‡ "Breastfeeding Disparities Exist," Breastfeeding Facts, CDC, accessed June 15, 2022, https://www.cdc.gov/breastfeeding/data/facts.html.

us dying or struggling to parent our children in ways of abundance versus ways of survival. It's one thing to be informed about BIPOC disparities and assist in creating more understanding and safety for Black people. It's another thing to perpetuate disparities by focusing on the harsh realities (or consequences) of inequity without moving into action, and by not also speaking to the ways BIPOC communities have continued to survive and thrive with the ongoing threat of racism and discrimination throughout the many systems we interact with. We would all benefit from those places also highlighting why these statistics are what they are, the work that BIPOC communities have been doing to combat this, how these organizations are planning to change these statistics, how they are holding individuals and organizations accountable, and what the consequences of the continued violence against Black birthing people will be.

Though we are years away from the events and people mentioned in the previous chapter, I also want to mention that managing your expectations will be very important in this next chapter. In some ways, things have changed—and in some ways, they have not. For example, we spoke about Black midwives in Alabama, with one of the last legally practicing Black midwives, Onnie Lee Logan, closing her practice in 1984 after lay midwives were outlawed in 1976. Alabama did not allow midwives to practice again until 2017, and the first five Alabama out-of-hospital midwives were licensed on January 19, 2019.* Stephanie Mitchell became the first Black licensed out-of-hospital midwife in Alabama in 2020. She also is the owner of the Birth Sanctuary Gainesville, the first freestanding birthing center in Alabama, providing trauma-informed and affirming care to all birthing people. It pains me to think about the current Alabama Black

---

* Anna Claire Vollers, "Midwives Can Legally Deliver Alabama Babies for First Time in Decades as State Issues Licenses," *AL*, January 19, 2019, https://www.al.com/news/2019/01/midwives-can-legally-deliver-alabama-babies-for-first-time-in-decades-as-state-issues-licenses.html.

perinatal death disparity (Black birthing people die at 2.5 times the rate of white birthing people in this state)* and its connection to out-of-hospital midwives being outlawed until fairly recently.

In a conversation I had with Stephanie Mitchell, she points out that it's important to remember, "when we think about statistics and how records were kept [from the 1930s through the Jim Crow era], statistics for what would be described in the literature as the 'negro people' were not even tabulated. As the timeline moves along, the statistics were sharpened, especially after the eradication of the midwife. The United States has done a better job in keeping hold of statistics, but it's been a system that is consistently problematic. In these statistics, what we're looking to see is that now we've shifted the health care of the pregnant individual from out of the home and out of the care of these problematic, vulturous midwives and into the hands of the hospitals that are supposed to be prestigious and medically advanced, what do the statistics say? You would like to see an improvement. However, it's not that we've seen no change—what in fact has happened is we've seen a worsening of statistics. And that should spark the attention of individuals. But the maternal care system has not changed . . . there has been no drastic overhaul. So you're not going to see the improvement that you seek; you're going to see a worsening of statistics until there is a systematic overhaul of the reasons why this is happening, which is not any biological factor of what it means to exist in a Black body, as opposed to any other body."[†]

I'll pose the question to you that I also asked myself after speaking with Mitchell: Is the present state of Black perinatal health much different from its past iterations? In my opinion, there has been

---

* "Racial Disparities," Save Alabama Moms, *Alabama Medicine*, accessed June 15, 2022, https://alabamamedicine.org/savealmoms/#1574279800496-da6debc5-5990.

† Stephanie Mitchell (@doctor_midwife), "Getting Right to the RJ Shits w/ @doctor _midwife," Instagram live @sabia_wade, filmed April 18, 2022, https://www.instagram.com/p/CcgHyuKJuav/.

improvement on recording what is happening to Black birthing bodies, but we still have a long way to go on improving the outcomes in a way that aligns with the ever-increasing technology and knowledge we have. The work, in some ways, is just beginning.

In this chapter we will be discussing present-day perspectives and the racial divide, so I want to mention a few things before we move forward. It is one thing to talk about history (something we all feel removed from), but as we move into this conversation about the reality of today, the intensity of this may feel different to you mentally, physically, and spiritually because there is no disconnection available. This is the here and now.

BIPOC people—I value your attentiveness to this chapter and ask you to notice any signs and symptoms of overwhelm you may be experiencing. You and your ancestors have done the labor continuously, so this space is made for you to consume this information in a way that is in rhythm with your needs. You have the permission to feel, to stop, to continue all at your own pace.

Non-BIPOC people—I also value your attentiveness to this chapter and ask you to notice any signs or symptoms that may be related to overwhelm, denial, fear, and other emotions that may come up for you. However, my bigger ask of you is different from my ask of BIPOC folks. I ask you to sit with those feelings and sensations, see those feelings through to the other side. I am ultimately asking you to build capacity for discomfort, something that culturally the non-BIPOC community is missing. You may have to pause, breathe, move, write, run, or do whatever is needed to help you see these emotions and sensations through, but do not avoid them or try to cope by pushing them away. Remember, you are here to do the work.

Last note as we continue through this chapter: I will not be repeating the statistics over and over again because we are more than numbers and bars on a graph. We are people. People who have continued to deal with our bodies being brutalized, commodified, and devalued all in one breath while being tasked with fixing a system that we didn't create.

Current Disparities (Perinatal, Infant, Lactation) and Connection Between Outcomes (such as SIDS and Lack of Black Providers)

In the last five years, I have noticed a big shift in bringing attention to Black perinatal and infant health disparities in the United States. These disparities aren't new, even though the hyperfocus across media makes it seem so. In the years of enslavement, slaveholders and physicians began to focus highly on the continuous reproduction of Black children, especially when the transatlantic slave trade became illegal in 1807–1808. As I've mentioned before, Black midwives would take care of their community members, but when the transatlantic slave trade became illegal, the system of slavery depended on the reproduction of Black children to continue. White physicians began to focus on Black childbirth and began recording the high infant mortality rates, blaming Black birthing people and midwives but not taking into account their own lack of training or knowledge of the childbirth process. At this time, half of the infants born into slavery were reported to have died within one year of their birth.*

As we look at statistics in our present time, they show Black birthing people and their infants are still at a higher risk of dying than non-BIPOC birthing people, even with the benefits of modern medicine and technology.

Why is that?

Many hypothesized that the Black perinatal and infant health disparities were caused by factors such as education, socioeconomic

---

* Deirdre Cooper Owens and Sharla M. Fett, "Black Maternal and Infant Health: Historical Legacies of Slavery," *American Journal of Public Health* 109, no. 10 (October 2019): 1342–1345, doi: 10.2105/AJPH.2019.305243, 1343.

status, health, access to health care, and employment status. Studies throughout the 1980s and 1990s set out to test these factors in an attempt to gain a better understanding of the root cause and create a plan of action to literally save the lives of Black birthing people and infants.

> In the 1980s, health officials began focusing on access to prenatal care as a way to reduce these perceived risk factors. The result, said Dr. Michael Lu, an ob-gyn and leading infant-mortality researcher, was more women getting care, but little improvement in birth outcomes. Instead, the racial gap grew. Black women who received prenatal care starting in the first trimester were still losing children at higher rates than white women who never saw a doctor during their pregnancies.[*]

Multiple studies, including the 2017 study named "Implicit Bias in Healthcare Professionals: A Systematic Review," concluded that the reason for these disparities was racism and discrimination in the health care system. Every attempt to control and increase factors, such as immediate prenatal care for Black birthing people, continued to not show any significant effects to the Black perinatal and infant mortality rates.[†]

This information has also forced the medical field to think about the ways Black birthing people are blamed for their outcomes instead of placing the blame on the medical system and practitioners caring for Black birthing people. For example, how many of us have heard that Black birthing people struggle with pregnancy complications such

---

[*] Zoë Carpenter, "What's Killing America's Black Infants?," *The Nation*, February 15, 2017, https://www.thenation.com/article/archive/whats-killing-americas-black-infants/.

[†] Chloë FitzGerald and Samia Hurst, "Implicit Bias in Healthcare Professionals: A Systematic Review," *BMC Medical Ethics* 18, no. 1 (2017): 19, doi: 10.1186/s12910-017-0179-8.

as preeclampsia and gestational diabetes, as if the birthing person's habits are the reason for their demise? Instead, information from these studies shows that the stress and trauma of being a Black birthing person in the United States who is constantly involved in racial and discriminatory systems has a major and sometimes deadly effect on Black birthing people and our children. This phenomenon has a name: *weathering*.

Weathering is defined as the process of wearing or being worn by long exposure to the atmosphere. In this context, weathering speaks to the long-term biological and psychological effects for birthing people of dealing with constant and long-term stressors in their environments within Black communities. These stressors include everything from microaggressions to the historically unfair treatment and trauma Black people have faced generationally in systems such as the criminal justice system and education systems.*

As a doula serving all communities in San Diego, I often found myself seeing stark differences in my Black and white clients who seemingly had similar lives from an external perspective. For example, I had a non-BIPOC client, a former nurse, expecting her second child with her husband, a physician. Her pregnancy was healthy, and her birth was a planned hospital birth. During our prenatals, we went over her birth plan, and she expressed generally feeling safe in the care of her ob-gyn and the hospital staff during the labor process. She had some worries about balancing a household of two children with her husband having to be away at times, so she also hired me to be her postpartum doula, along with her current sitter who assisted with her older child. She felt financially secure and had no barriers to accessing doula care or any additional resources not provided by her health insurance, such as the pelvic floor therapy she regularly attended.

---

* Arline T. Geronimus et al., "'Weathering' and Age Patterns of Allostatic Load Scores Among Blacks and Whites in the United States," *American Journal of Public Health* 96, no. 5 (May 2006): 826–833.

Similarly, I had a Black client, located in San Diego, at the time expecting her second child as well. She was a single parent with an active toddler, her family was unfortunately not local to assist her, and she did not have the financial ability to hire a sitter. She did have a partner, but he was long distance and had plans to fly in to be by her side during the birthing process and for a couple weeks after, meaning she would be on her own within a couple weeks of having her child. She was living in a small apartment in a not-so-safe area and was also working full time but highly stressed over her current cost of living and the expenses that come with a newborn. During our prenatal visits, she shared her plan to have a hospital birth but also expressed not feeling safe or confident in the hospital system because of the Black perinatal and infant disparities. Cost of doula care was a barrier for her, but I was able to provide her with a discounted price because I understood the literal need for my assistance during such a vulnerable time in her life. Her mind and body were consistently stressed with the daily struggle of living, as well as with carrying the load of what it means to be a Black person in this world, when she should have been able to focus on herself during her pregnancy and have the support to allow her mental and physical health to thrive. Instead, her experience was clouded with fear of discrimination, racism, and constant struggle as systems continued to fail her despite her efforts to succeed.

For those who are unaware, allow me catch you up to speed with some of the current stressors currently impacting Black communities:

- 1 in 11 Black adults are currently under correctional control (in prison or on parole/probation).
- 1 in 230 Black youth are detained in juvenile facilities.
- 1 in 1,000 Black men and boys will die at the hands of police.
- 1 in 3 Black families have zero or negative wealth.

- 1 in 2.5 Black adults were unemployed or temporarily furloughed in April 2020.
- 1 in 4 Black children born in 1990 will experience their father in prison in their lifetime.
- 1 in 6.5 Black children have elevated lead levels in their blood.
- 1 in 7 Black children suffer from asthma.*

Pause and read those statistics again. Slowly this time. Add in faces of the Black people in your families and in your communities. Take notice of how these statistics show a broad view of what to expect in your life as a Black person in the United States: more interactions with the criminal justice system, increased health issues beginning at an early age, lack of unemployment, police violence, broken families, and a lack of wealth. This is only a small reflection of what Black birthing people are weighed down with, generationally and daily.

Somatic Exercise: The Weight of Stress

How did it feel to read the statistics above about the many experiences Black people are having while trying to navigate their lives? Just in these statistics we can see how Black people have a higher risk of everything from asthma to being incarcerated, as well as not being able to create wealth, all factors contributing to the quality of their lives. What sensations ran through your body as you moved through each statistic? Did you feel nothing or numb because it's not an experience you could relate to? No answer is wrong, but it is important that we all push ourselves into feeling the heaviness of not being deprioritized, not as a way to traumatize but in a way to relate or at least try to understand. For many of

* Hedwig Lee et al., "The Demographics of Racial Inequality in the United States," Brookings, July 27, 2020, https://www.brookings.edu/blog/up-front/2020/07/27/the-demographics-of-racial-inequality-in-the-united-states/.

you, especially non-BIPOC people or people with many privileged identities, it may be hard to understand the weight of stress, but in this next exercise we will aim to feel just a small portion of what many BIPOC individuals feel every day.

Let's begin by imagining a time when you felt relatively good about yourself. Maybe it was one day when you accomplished a goal at work, or maybe it was when you got through a challenging part of your life. What did it feel like to feel good? What sensations did you feel (e.g., open heart, buzzing energy throughout your body, literal lightness in your feet)? What emotions did you feel (e.g., happiness, pride, excitement, satisfaction)? Take it all in and allow yourself to be physically and emotionally back in that moment as if it were happening right this very moment.

Now imagine that in the moment of feeling positive and proud of yourself someone with authority or even someone you closely care about begins to tell you, "You aren't enough. You are a threat to society. You will have a harder time obtaining your goals no matter what path you choose. You will struggle, especially if you do not conform to my rules and push your own culture further away. You will have to work twice as hard to get to where I am, and even that is not promised." What do you feel right now? Are you still feeling that sense of pride and joy?

As this person continues to badger you, you ask the simple question of why, and their response is "Because of the color of your skin." How does it feel to know that for a reason completely out of your control your life would be negatively affected? That even if you tried hard and did everything nearly perfectly, you would still have to deal with issues others do not face? This is the experience of BIPOC people living in the world, striving to take care of themselves and their families but historically being deprioritized and punished for no other reason than the color of their skin. Please allow yourself to pause and ride the wave of the emotions that come up for you, as well as write down any thoughts or feelings coming up for you in your journal.

When we look at this information, we now can begin to reframe our questions from "How do we help Black birthing people to live longer?" to "How do we change the systems that have caused these disparities, and change them permanently and for many lifetimes to come?" Remembering that Black birthing people are not the cause of these disparities and are instead the victims of these systems that continue to perpetuate harm with little to no accountability.

Black Communities and Weathering: The Physical and Mental Impact on Black Bodies

We've discussed the impact that weathering has on perinatal health, but another important disparity caused by weathering is the heightened rate of Black infant mortality. According to the CDC, the top five reasons for infant mortality are as follows:*

1. Birth defects
2. Preterm birth and low birth weight
3. Injuries (e.g., suffocation)
4. Sudden Infant Death Syndrome (SIDS)
5. Maternal pregnancy complications

There are a few connections that I would like to make when mentioning these top five causes and their specific connection to Black birthing people. First, let's note that the rates of lactation in the Black

---

* "Causes of Infant Mortality," Infant Mortality, CDC, accessed June 15, 2022, https://www.cdc.gov/reproductivehealth/maternalinfanthealth/infantmortality.htm.

community are lower than in any other racial group in the United States. Next, the injuries mentioned in category three are something we don't always have the ability to control, even though I'm sure there are some avoidable injuries within that category. However, when we relate the other disparities to weathering, we must ask: If the racism and discrimination in the systems we currently maneuver in were to decrease or be eliminated, would the rates of birth defects, preterm births and low birth weight, and perinatal complication caused by ongoing stress and trauma decrease significantly? That is a big question and not one that we can easily figure out, but there is one factor that can be tested and affected positively—and that is the fourth top cause of infant mortality death: Sudden Infant Death Syndrome.

Sudden Infant Death Syndrome, commonly referred to as SIDS, is the sudden, unexplained death of a healthy-presenting baby that typically occurs while the baby is asleep. "While the cause of SIDS is unknown, many clinicians and researchers believe that SIDS is associated with problems in the ability of the baby to arouse from sleep, to detect low levels of oxygen, or a buildup of carbon dioxide in the blood."[*]

In a study titled "Does Breastfeeding Reduce the Risk of Sudden Infant Death Syndrome?" released in March 2009, research indicated that bodyfeeding during infancy decreased the risk of SIDS by approximately half.[†] Another study, in 2017, showed that the risk of SIDS was decreased by half with a bodyfeeding duration of at least two months. It also concluded that exclusive bodyfeeding isn't necessary to offer this protection—a combination of formula and bodyfeeding provides protections to the infant as well.[‡]

---

[*] "What You Need to Know About SIDS," Sudden Infant Death Syndrome (SIDS), Children's Hospital, accessed June 15, 2022, https://www.childrenshospital.org/conditions/sudden-infant-death-syndrome-sids.

[†] M. Vennemann et al., "Does Breastfeeding Reduce the Risk of Sudden Infant Death Syndrome?," *Pediatrics* 123, no. 3 (2009): 406–10, doi: 10.1542.

[‡] John Thompson et al., "Duration of Breastfeeding and Risk of SIDS: An Individual Participant Data Meta-Analysis," *Pediatrics* 140 (2017), https://doi.org/10.1542/peds.2017-1324.

These studies along with others have proven that bodyfeeding can assist with decreasing infant mortality—however, it is important not to frame Black birthing people as *choosing* not to bodyfeed and think about what barriers are being placed in front of Black birthing people who are wanting to feed their babies human milk.

We will focus on the following barriers that currently exist for Black birthing people seeking and desiring to bodyfeed: racism, lack of inclusion, accessibility, the commercialization and commodification of lactation, an absence of culturally humble care, and generational trauma.

Racism in Lactation

When thinking about racism and bodyfeeding, it's easy to connect to the idea of obviously racist practitioners discouraging bodyfeeding and withholding resources for Black birthing people, but I challenge you to go deeper than that. Much of the racism that exists in bodyfeeding is also implicit, or not particularly conscious or obvious. For example, "Black moms in the Special Supplemental Nutrition Program for Women, Infants, and Children (WIC) are less likely to receive breastfeeding counseling than white mothers in the same program."[*] This fact contributes to the current widespread belief throughout the professional birth community that Black birthing people are generally more interested in formula feeding their children, which is simply not true. It is true that many Black birthing people share many ideas of whether they would prefer to bodyfeed or formula feed their child, and either choice is not wrong. However, a general assumption about Black birthing people preferring formula to human milk has led to Black birthing people not receiving necessary information, resources, and supplies to make a truly informed

* Claire Gillespie, "How Systemic Racism Contributes to Less Breastfeeding Amongst Black Mothers," Family and Parenting News, *Very Well Family*, February 24, 2021, https://www.verywellfamily.com/why-are-black-women-less-likely-to-breastfeed-5113076.

decision about their infant feeding choices, and if a choice is not informed, then it is not truly a choice.

I want to emphasize that formula itself is not a bad tool. It has become a lifesaving tool for many babies and has provided a form of relief for birthing parents all over the world. However, to understand the lower rates of bodyfeeding and high rates of formula used in the Black community, we must understand the origins of this connection. In her book *Skimmed*, Andrea Freeman shares the story of Annie Mae Fultz. Annie, a deaf Black-Cherokee mother of six children, had the world's first-recorded identical quadruplets on May 23, 1946. The girls were thriving and gaining fame as they continued to beat the odds. Fred Klenner, a non-BIPOC doctor, delivered the quadruplets, and as the girls gained fame, he decided to use their celebrity to bring attention to himself and his controversial theories. He began injecting the girls with doses of vitamin C and took it upon himself to name the children himself. He named all of them Mary and gave them the middle names of women relatives in his life, Ann, Louise, Alice, and Catherine. Next, Klenner decided to create a corporate partnership with a formula company, and the highest bid would be the first to target Black women with a formula advertising campaign featuring the Fultz Quad's success story. St. Louis's PET Milk Company was selected, and so began the chain of events that led to formula being strategically pushed to Black families, as well as Annie Mae losing the rights to her own children. The campaign created high profits for PET Milk and the company was the first to see such high numbers without marketing beauty products, alcohol, or tobacco to Black families. PET Milk's marketing convinced Black parents that formula was as healthy as, if not healthier than, human milk, which provided comfort and convenience for Black parents dealing with and seeking relief from the external pressures of bodyfeeding, such as cost, education, access, and stigma. Although PET Milk's marketing strategy was incorrect and deceptive, the effects of these actions can still be felt today, especially in the way Black images are highly exploited to market formula use but not seen nearly as much in promoting positive imaging of bodyfeeding. PET Milk's strategic marketing also created and propelled the image of Black birthing people choosing to use formula to feed their children as the superior and "right" choice, making them "good" parents—either consciously or subconsciously—in the eyes of people engaging with these parents, especially birth professionals.*

There is also another aspect to this ongoing conversation about racism in bodyfeeding, and that is the lack of Black practitioners in the lactation field. For example, International Board Certified Lactation Consultants (IBCLC) are the highest accredited health care professional specializing in lactation support for birthing people. IBCLCs assist birthing people by providing education and assisting with common difficulties such as low milk supply, pain with lactation, infants with tongue and lip ties, infant weight gain, and conditions like mastitis. IBCLCs often support birthing parents in their homes and in their communities, centering access and assisting parents with their lactation journey as much as possible. However, "it is believed that less than 2% of IBCLCs are Black or African-American" in the United States.† This lack of Black IBCLCs who could be out in their communities increasing bodyfeeding rates is not due to a lack of interest but from a host of barriers to this education, including cost, accessing loans, location of programs, time to complete the program, ability to complete internship, and being in systems that do not provide ongoing support for Black students in IBCLC programs. This example of IBCLCs is only one of many demonstrating how racism is affecting

* Andrea Freeman, *Skimmed: Breastfeeding, Race, and Injustice* (Stanford, CA: Stanford University Press, 2020), chapter 1.
† Janiya M. Williams, "Disrupting Disparities & Exclusion in Lactation," National Committee for Responsive Philanthropy, September 16, 2021, https://www.ncrp.org/2021/09/disrupting-lactation-disparities.html.

the accessibility to create more Black practitioners for Black birthing people and their communities.

Lack of Inclusion

Notice that I am using the term *bodyfeeding* when referring to the process of providing human milk to an infant. *Bodyfeeding* and *chestfeeding* are terminology choices that can be used to be inclusive of trans and nonbinary folks who may want to use a term that feels more in alignment with their relationship to their body and lactation. I will be using *bodyfeeding* to describe lactation for all bodies. Queer and trans Black birthing people exist, and many are aiming to be active participants in their lactation journey but are not finding resources that center or even acknowledge their existence. Queer and trans birthing people create their families in different ways and deserve to have their experiences talked about in a way that can provide assistance and encouragement during their lactation journey. For example, a Black trans birthing parent may want to bodyfeed their child and may be interested in induced lactation but be unable to find resources to gain this information or any safe trans-affirming groups to sit in community with. When this happens, and it happens often, this is a missed opportunity for the birthing parent, their child, and their overall family. When thinking about your exposure to bodyfeeding resources (classes, websites, books, etc.), how many of these spaces utilize inclusive language? I can safely assume not many. When inclusive language is not used, many people's experiences are erased, and necessary opportunities to encourage and support bodyfeeding are made unavailable and inaccessible, contributing to a lower potential to increase bodyfeeding journeys. I also want to emphasize that inclusion doesn't stop at rainbow flags, pronouns, inclusive language, and learning about the methods that can be utilized to assist in lactation for queer and trans birthing people. It also means creating supportive places through setting standards and expectations for respecting the differences of everyone in the community, as well as ways to deal with nuance and inevitable rupture and repair in these spaces.

Accessibility

In 2010 the Affordable Care Act included the amended section 7 of the Fair Labor Standard Act (FLSA) requiring employers to "provide a reasonable break time" for birthing parents expressing milk after the birth of a child. The amendment also requires the employer to provide an adequate space to express milk, "a place, other than a bathroom, that is shielded from view and free from intrusion from coworkers and the public."* These protections are valid for a year after giving birth, and the employer is not required to provide compensation for these breaks or any time spent toward the purpose of expressing milk. These federal regulations cannot be enforced if an employer has fewer than fifty employees or the requirements "impose an undue burden" on the employer.† Although these regulations were meant to create an added layer of protection for lactating parents, it left many parents out of the equation. Many lactating parents, often low-income BIPOC parents, work for smaller companies that are not required to follow these regulations, which then leaves them with the burden of figuring out how to express milk during a long shift without proper breaks or a clean location for themselves and their lactation supplies. I have heard many stories of parents expressing their milk in public bathrooms, becoming painfully engorged due to lack of proper breaks, and sometimes even dealing with plugged ducts and severe mastitis as a result of not being able to express their

---

* Department of Labor, "Fact Sheet #73: Break Time for Nursing Mothers under the FSLA," Wage and hour division, DOL, accessed June 15, 2022, https://www.dol.gov/agencies/whd/fact-sheets/73-flsa-break-time-nursing-mothers.

† "Section 7(r) of the Fair Labor Standards Act," Wage and Hour Division, DOL, accessed June 15, 2022, https://www.dol.gov/agencies/whd/nursing-mothers/law.

milk properly for their child. There are also many mental effects to not having the ability to express milk properly, such as depression, anxiety, and an overall feeling that they are not a good parent because of the daily circumstances and stress involved with trying to feed their child human milk. These pressures and complications have led to many lactating parents deciding to feed their child with formula and let their supply dry up before they are physically or mentally ready. Unfortunately, these experiences are also vastly connected to only some lactating parents having access to the Family Medical Leave Act (FMLA) in the United States. For certain covered employees, FMLA provides up to twelve weeks of paid parental leave for the birth of a baby or the adoptive or foster placement of a child. To qualify for paid parental leave, the employee should have been employed by the same employer for the last year, with a minimum of 1,250 hours of work. The company must also have more than fifty employees within a seventy-five mile range.* Once again, parents who do not qualify (and many do not) are left to figure out how they will financially support themselves and their family after the birth of their child. Some parents may have a partner or family members that can financially assist them, but many are forced to return to work weeks, and often days, after giving birth. The unfortunate immediate return to work does not allow the postpartum body to heal properly, and often the choice to bodyfeed is untenable during this time.

The importance of accessibility became even more apparent during "The Great Formula Shortage" of 2021. The cause of the formula shortage included formula recalls, supply disruption, and legislation, but the impact of the formula shortage was felt by all, especially BIPOC communities. The immediate and dangerous impact of this shortage was infants being unable to receive the vital nutrition they need and

---

* "Frequently Asked Questions and Answers About the Revisions to the Family and Medical Leave Act," Wage and Hour Division, DOL, accessed June 15, 2022, https://www.dol.gov/agencies/whd/fmla/final-rule/faq.

parents seeking alternative (and sometimes unsafe) practices such as making their own formula to feed their infants. Another result of this shortage was people buying formula in bulk in order to hoard a supply until the shortage ends, as well as formula being resold at astronomical prices because the demand for the formula is so high. Black and Latinx birthing parents were affected by this shortage greatly due to having lower lactation rates and lower income, leaving many Black and Latinx birthing parents unable to buy formula in bulk and at the higher prices for the formula that remained available. Many Black and Latinx birthing parents are aiming to lactate more or relactate, but their accessibility to lactation support services is not nearly as robust as needed. In response to this formula shortage, the government slightly eased current laws that make it difficult to access formula internationally, but more privileged communities gained access to these shipments before low-income Black and Latinx communities. Lastly, "breastfeeding is free" rhetoric was thrown around, when the truth is, there is a cost associated with bodyfeeding, which includes the cost of supplies, pumps, education, lactation consultants, etc. Accessibility matters, and in this case, lack of accessibility may be the literal cause of death or complications for many infants.

The Commercialization and Commodification of Lactation

Birthing bodies, especially Black birthing bodies, have often been seen as a monetized asset by the medical-industrial complex, and this fact does not stop when it comes to the monetization of lactation. Take a moment to think about the imagery you have seen for bodyfeeding advertising across platforms such as websites, pamphlets, books, and videos. Do you see many images of BIPOC bodyfeeding parents, or is that imagery mostly of those with privileged identities, such as non-BIPOC, thin, cis women? This lack of imagery is only a part of the problem, but it creates a conscious and unconscious thought that bodyfeeding is predominantly a non-BIPOC activity and highly connected to the strategy to connect Black imagery to formula feeding and non-BIPOC imagery to bodyfeeding. Furthermore, bodyfeeding has been complicated by the message that to bodyfeed requires many supplies, from top-quality breast pumps that cost hundreds of dollars to name-brand pillows that cost way more than many people can afford. To be clear, not every bodyfeeding journey is simple, and many journeys may require additional supplies—but the cost of these supplies can be inaccessible to many and discouraging, to say the least, leading to BIPOC birthing people defaulting to formula feeding. I have often experienced prenatal clients who either have been gifted or have purchased many nursing-related items before their child was born because they have been inundated with the message of being prepared for any and all bodyfeeding possibilities. Often after purchasing these items, they later experience feeling as if they spent money on items they never used or the baby didn't like—and even experience guilt from spending money that could have been saved or used for additional items. I aim to relieve that guilt by explaining to clients that they, along with other parents, are immersed in messaging that equates good parenting with buying the most expensive supplies, and lots of them. In the 2020 study "Commercialisation and Commodification of Breastfeeding: Video Diaries by First-Time Mothers," researchers found that "women preparing for breastfeeding are exposed to increasing commercialisation. When things do not go to plan, women are even more exposed to commercial solutions. The impact of online marketing strategies fueled their need for paraphernalia so that their dependence on such items became important aspects of their parenting and breastfeeding experiences."*

---

* Alison M. Taylor et al., "Commercialisation and Commodification of Breastfeeding: Video Diaries by First-Time Mothers," *International Breastfeeding Journal* 15, no. 33 (2020): 1, https://doi.org/10.1186/s13006-020-00264-1.

It is important to remember that tools to assist in supporting and extending a birthing person's lactation journey can be helpful, but the commercialization and commodification of lactation can create barriers and inaccessibility for marginalized communities, especially BIPOC birthing parents.

Culturally Humble Care

Before we move further, let's talk about the difference between *cultural competence* and *cultural humility*. Cultural competence is the socialized, learned approach of accepting differences and being able to interact with others. Cultural humility is a lifelong practice of self-awareness (including awareness of biases) that is oriented toward interpersonal connection. Cultural competence assumes that there's an end point to learning about someone's identity and ways of existing, whereas cultural humility invites the participant to build an ongoing practice of learning identities and ways people exist in order to create stronger interpersonal relationships. An example of this would be a non-BIPOC lactation consultant assuming a Black person does not want to bodyfeed due to generational trauma based on a literature they have read (cultural competence), which could be true but is not every Black person's story, versus a non-BIPOC lactation consultant learning about the history of Black lactation and asking their Black client their personal reasons for not wanting to bodyfeed (cultural humility). Simply put, cultural competence can be desired and learned for purely capitalistic reasons without any real internal growth, but cultural humility places the power in the client's hand and creates a collaborative approach to care, which benefits everyone involved.

Caring for birthing people is never one size fits all. When it comes to bodyfeeding, it can be a very complicated decision to make and include factors such as culture, location, familial history, trauma, income, and more. Having culturally humble providers offering support during this time is very important for the birthing person. Being understood and heard is vital to creating an environment that allows a birthing person to explore the possibilities around bodyfeeding, as well as the barriers they may come against and the fears or hesitation they may have. For example, I began working as a postpartum doula with a Black client with a beautiful new set of one-month-old twin girls. She was struggling with the balancing act of having twins but was very excited about the possibilities of bodyfeeding, even though she was mostly using formula to feed her children. During our first time together, I asked her about her bodyfeeding journey and if there was anything I could do to assist her in producing more human milk for children. Through that conversation, I learned she was interested in producing more human milk but did not feel educated enough on how to do so. She expressed that most of her care team throughout the pregnancy were non-BIPOC people. Many of them gave her resources and directed her to lactation classes to attend, but when she attended those classes, she was often the only Black person, and also felt that she was the only low-income parent in the space. Although the intentions of the class were to be helpful, she left feeling isolated and unable to afford or access the resources being offered in the class, which eventually led to her accepting that bodyfeeding wasn't going to be a part of her parenting. Being Black myself, I validated her experience and empathized with her greatly. From there I assisted her with culturally humble education that helped her to produce human milk for her children while also supporting her in finding low-cost items in her community and utilizing tools she already had at home, like the simplicity of folding a couple pillows to assist her in supporting her while bodyfeeding instead of encouraging her to buy a single-purpose thirty-dollar pillow she could not afford. Culturally humble care increases trust and safety, improves communication, promotes inclusion, increases community engagement, and closes care gaps by providing appropriate resources.

Generational Trauma

Last but not least, history cannot be missed in this conversation of bodyfeeding for Black birthing people. During times of slavery and beyond, Black women were used as wet nurses for white families. Traditionally a wet nurse was a woman who bodyfed and cared for another family's child. For Black birthing people of the time, this position was involuntary or a means of survival for themselves and their families. Enslaved Black wet nurses were given the task of feeding the descendants of the very people who held them captive, demeaned them, and thought of them as property and not people. Many non-BIPOC birthing people felt nursing was not supportive of their lifestyle because it kept them from being able to wear the trendy clothes of the times. The solution to this was forcing Black slaves into doing the work of feeding the non-BIPOC children from their enslaved bodies. Their bodies were also thought to provide natural immunity from malaria to these non-BIPOC children, as malaria was a top killer of white settlers at the time.

One of the many downfalls to wet nursing, besides being forced into doing so, was that Black mothers were not allowed to feed their own children with their human milk. Instead Black babies drank cow and goat milk, which led to higher mortality in Black children who weren't protected from diseases that they would have gained increased immunity from through human milk. Wet nursing also created a large gap in the Black family, as Black enslaved wet nurses were unable to spend time with their own families because of their responsibility to be available at any time for the children of their enslavers. This history of wet nursing and the disconnection of Black parents from their children during a crucial period of nursing, immunization, and connection can still be felt in the Black community generations later.*

---

* Kamna Kirti, "The Tragic Plight of Enslaved Wet Nurses: How Black Mothers Were Systematically Deprived of Breastfeeding Their Own Children," *Lessons*

All these factors contribute to the ability—or lack thereof—of Black birthing people to bodyfeed their children. It is a decision that is very layered, nuanced, and filled with barriers that non-BIPOC people are historically not faced with at the level Black people are. When non-BIPOC are faced with similar factors, research shows there are more resources available to get through and overcome these barriers. With all these barriers and hardships to bodyfeeding for Black birthing people, are Black birthing people *really* able to have a true choice in the matter of bodyfeeding? The reality is some Black birthing people, especially those with intersecting oppressions such as being low income, disabled, working beyond full-time hours, etc., are often not given the choice to bodyfeed and are instead pushed into formula feeding because they do not have any support or resources that would allow them to bodyfeed their child successfully. Bodyfeeding, a natural occurrence that some people may want to do but feel is out of reach, has become a privilege due to the systems and barriers in place to maintain low bodyfeeding rates and higher formula feeding rates for Black birthing parents. In order for that privilege to be an actual option and choice for everyone, many systems would have to change, from educational systems that are currently upholding barriers for BIPOC people wanting to work within the lactation field to the federal government that currently only allows certain people to receive paid parental leave and have time and space to express milk at their place of employment. This is why the work of collective liberation is necessary to not only overhaul systems but also to connect people to the humanness of all of our experiences beyond these systems. We need and deserve more.

As Freeman says in *Skimmed,*

---

from History, Medium, August 2, 2020, https://medium.com/lessons-from-history /the-tragic-plight-of-enslaved-wet-nurses-b1c80b73f290.

But it is so hidden by the fact that we think of breastfeeding as a very intimate and personal choice, when in fact, for many people, there is no choice at all. And that is due directly to the acts of the government through law, through policy, through partnership with the formula industry. So I think racial justice needs to incorporate these hidden oppressions that pretend that we're just making choices based on personal preferences, when in fact, we're all just responding to our circumstances that are set by forces greater than us.*

Lactivist

Lactivism is a specific form of activism focused on not only promoting bodyfeeding but also addressing systemic inequities, as well as advocating for underprivileged communities aiming to increase bodyfeeding. Inclusive lactivism doesn't discriminate and is inclusive of the full spectrum of birthing people, as well as the full spectrum of infant feeding choices, including formula feeding. Lactivism has become a crucial part of implementing and promoting change on a larger scale but also, and more important, creating resources for underprivileged communities needing assistance immediately.

Jarrah Foster is a Black International Board Certified Lactation Consultant (IBCLC) and the owner of Lactation & Wellness in San Diego, California. Foster has a host of services, from assisting in human milk supply and baby positioning to assessments of oral latching. She also offers appreciative coaching, a form of support that utilizes positive reinforcement and emotional attunement to increase self-efficacy, bonding, and attachment between parent and baby while

---

* Andrea Freeman, "From Breastfeeding to Beyoncé, 'Skimmed' Tells a New Story About Black Motherhood," interview by Breandrea July, Public Health, *NPR*, February 11, 2020, https://www.npr.org/sections/health-shots/2020/02/11/801343800/from-breastfeeding-to-beyonc-skimmed-tells-a-new-story-about-black-motherhood.

encouraging mindfulness and enjoyment of the experience. Foster is one of very few Black IBCLCs in Southern California and has made a great impact on many different community members by creating culturally humble and accessible care.

Stephanie Brown, also an IBCLC and a reproductive health advocate, is located in Philadelphia and has been a guest educator at Birthing Advocacy Doula Trainings for several cohorts. Stephanie offers group and one-on-one consulting with an emphasis on queer- and trans-competent care. Stephanie's approach to birth work creates a space for *every* body and promotes the ongoing support that is needed for parents who may have particular needs that are usually not addressed in mainstream health care.

Nurturely, a nonprofit based in Eugene, Oregon, is on a mission to promote equity in perinatal wellness and strengthen cultures of support for infants and caregivers through preventative knowledge-sharing, collaborative exploration, and proactive community engagement. Nurturely provides services to both professionals and birthing people actively lactating or preparing to lactate. Nurturely supports birthing people by supporting and uplifting programs such as "Nurturing BLACK: Baby's Lived Experience as Cultural Kinship" created by Ayesha Elliot, a mentorship series for non-BIPOC expectant parents raising Black or biracial babies. Nurturely's programming for professionals includes many educational opportunities, such as their annual Milk Mood Moves conference, "an interdisciplinary conference for health professionals, researchers, and advocates to share the latest science and clinical knowledge of pregnancy, birth, and postpartum, focusing on human milk and lactation, perinatal mood disorders, and physiology and biomechanics of the perinatal period."* Nurturely provides much of its programming in English and Spanish. It also has

---

* "Milk, Mood, Moves," Continuing Professional Development, School of Medicine at Oregon Health and Science University, accessed June 15, 2022, https://www.ohsu.edu /school-of-medicine/cpd/milk-mood-moves.

in-person and virtual support of babywearing and ongoing memorial spaces dedicated to lost babies for grieving birthing parents. Nurturely is an example of how to bridge the gap between birthing people and professionals through the goals of creating equitable structures to support the availability of lactation services and education for all.

Individual lactation educators and organizations are vital to the state of lactation in its present day. Without these individuals and organizations, many underserved communities would not have access to these resources and would not have the hands-on support needed to foster the lactation journey of BIPOC birthing parents. These individuals are currently working within a gap that has been created by privileged communities and broken systems that do not understand the true needs of BIPOC people aiming to bodyfeed while constantly battling systemic inequities.

4

REPRODUCTIVE JUSTICE AS THE PATH TO COLLECTIVE LIBERATION

If 60 percent of the deaths are preventable—and we have trainings, we have simulations that are going on in our hospitals in California and in the nation—it's not that we don't have the technology; we just lack the ability to see Black births and Black women as valuable.

—Karen A. Scott, associate professor of OB-GYN
and reproductive sciences, on panel "Black Mothers Matter:
Racism and Childbirth in America"

W E CAN THINK of reproductive justice in the same way we think about fixing our health care system. Right now, if you have something going on in your body, you go see your primary care physician. She figures out that it's something to do with your liver, so she gives you a referral to go to a hepatologist, who then sends you to a gastroenterologist, and so on and so forth. Often these strings of referrals—and the multiple doctor's appointments required for them that must be scheduled around work and childcare—are necessary for any insurance coverage of whatever is ailing the person. We treat the pieces of the body as separate entities, and few are connecting it all together.

Reproductive justice allows us to look at the whole picture. It's not just about having a safe birth. It's about whether the birthing person has the environmental, financial, and social support to have the family they want to have, when and how it works for them. It leads us to question whether a person has safe water to drink, whether their children can get a quality education, whether they have access to healthy food, and more. Reproductive justice doesn't just look at one small piece of racism—it looks at the whole puzzle. It is such a core aspect of collective liberation that it *is* in fact collective liberation: it is through reproductive justice that we can achieve true equity, inclusion, and autonomy.

Reproductive justice is a term that originated from Loretta Ross (a cofounder of SisterSong) and the Women of African Descent for Reproductive Justice. This group of Black women aimed to create reproductive justice as a framework that centered communities that were most marginalized. The creation of reproductive justice was a direct response to second-wave feminism in the 1960s to 1980s, which focused highly on improving the lives of non-BIPOC middle-class cis women and left many groups outside of those identities to fight for themselves or simply be forgotten. Second-wave feminism pushed issues such as the freedom to be safe regardless of sexuality, legal abortions, workplace equality, and marital rape. All these topics were and still are very important, but, for example, while non-BIPOC cis women were fighting for workplace equality, many BIPOC groups were fighting to even get into the workforce, and while non-BIPOC cis women were fighting for legal abortions, many BIPOC groups were fighting for basic health care access.

Reproductive justice has called in (not *out*) these truths by creating a framework that brought necessary attention to issues facing all people, especially marginalized communities such as BIPOC folks and trans people of color, such as comprehensive sex education, safe homes, access to contraception, and access to adequate health care, understanding that creating awareness for the most vulnerable would only have a positive ripple effect as change eventually affected all.

There are four pillars of reproductive justice, as outlined by SisterSong, an Atlanta based activist group committed to reproductive justice for women of color a national activist organization dedicated to reproductive justice for women of color. These pillars are foundational to the framework of reproductive justice and have been the anchor to the work I have done and continue to do:

To achieve reproductive justice, we must:

- Analyze power systems. Reproductive politics in the US is based on gendered, sexualized, and racialized acts of dominance that occur on a daily basis. RJ works to understand and eradicate these nuanced dynamics.
- Address intersecting oppressions. Audre Lorde said, "There is no such thing as a single-issue struggle because we do not live single-issue lives." Marginalized women face multiple oppressions, and we can only win freedom by addressing how they impact one another.

- Center the most marginalized. Our society will not be free until the most vulnerable people are able to access the resources and full human rights to live self-determined lives without fear, discrimination, or retaliation.
- Join together across issues and identities. All oppressions impact our reproductive lives; RJ is simply human rights seen through the lens of the nuanced ways oppression impacts self-determined family creation. The intersectionality of RJ is both an opportunity and a call to come together as one movement with the power to win freedom for all oppressed people.*

Analyzing Power Systems

What is a power system? Power systems are all around us. Initially your thought may be of the medical-industrial complex as a power system, which is true. However, I challenge you to become aware of power systems that even you take part in and the identities you carry that may increase your power. Usually those who are closer to power and have historically had more power are those with identities that have been valued and prioritized throughout American history—usually non-BIPOC, cisgendered, thin, neurotypical, financially stable people. That is not to say that BIPOC people cannot also have power, but that power is usually overshadowed and externally limited because of their racial identity, which cannot be hidden or changed. Remember, power is always present whether you are a doula or a doctor, a lactation consultant or someone with a specific experience, knowledge, or easy access to resources. In spaces where your experience, knowledge, or resources are more prevalent and evident in an interaction with an individual or group of people, you are deemed

* "Home Page: Goals," SisterSong, https://www.sistersong.net/.

as the more dominant or more powerful person in the interaction, which is a great responsibility. When we talk to our children, we are in power, and our power makes us responsible for what we say, how we say it, and the impact it has on the well-being of our children. When this responsibility is neglected or abused, our children become traumatized and unable to function as their greatest self. This is true of all powerful individuals and systems and the people in relationship with them.

So again, what is a power system? What power systems do we all participate in? I'm hoping that your answer has expanded to include medical, educational, and criminal justice systems as well as the different power systems in place that we are voluntarily or involuntarily pushed into participating within, which can include conversations we hold with community members every single day. These power systems and dynamics are particularly evident in the conversations about racism and its impact on Black birthing bodies. Currently, Black birthing people are dying in a medical system that was not built to protect them, but systems are communities of people. When thinking about the individuals and power dynamics within these systems that are interacting with Black birthing people, positions of power such as physicians and nurses come to mind. In those spaces, birth professionals can be of any race, but in the United States, non-BIPOC birth professionals are closer to power than their counterparts, meaning non-BIPOC birth professionals have a responsibility to engage their power while understanding that their actions, or inactions, will impact the well-being of Black birthing people navigating the health care system.

For non-BIPOC people, there are levels of moving toward owning responsibility of power and redistributing that power in a way that is led by the very people being harmed. The first level is to be a *white ally*, a term most people have some familiarity with. A white ally is a non-BIPOC person who believes in the goal of collective liberation by deconstructing white supremacy and systems that are currently in power. A white ally may spread the word of the current imbalances in the world but still be operating in their white privilege due to the passive nature of being an ally. Believing in equality and equity is not the same as actually doing something about it. That is where a *white accomplice* steps in. A white accomplice is a non-BIPOC person who takes action to effect change by helping marginalized communities create equitable, inclusive, and safe spaces, even if it negatively impacts the non-BIPOC person's own privilege or social standing. White accomplices are required to remove their ego, be led by voices that are often not heard, and trust that communities of color know what they need in order to thrive. White accomplices also understand the risk they are taking by actively opposing white supremacy and that the risk they are taking is only a fraction of the risk BIPOC individuals experience by just being themselves in a world that violates their safety and deprioritizes their existence. To be a white ally is the first step, but to be a white accomplice is the goal, and the only way to leverage power and privilege for the broader goal of collective liberation.

Let's go back to the birth room with Reena and Jarrod from chapter 1. Think about what power systems were present during this normal but unfortunate experience. For most of us, the first power system that comes to mind is the hospital system. Reena was having a baby in the American health care system. Some of the things that contributed to this huge power disparity were the hierarchy of medical practitioners (physicians, nurses, lactation consultants, nursing aides, etc.) and their levels of experience with childbirth, hospital policies that create rules and guidelines based on a "one size fits all" policy, fear of racism and discrimination by Reena and her family, the financial power of the hospital, medical forms that aren't easy to understand but have to be signed in order to receive medical assistance, and minimal to zero accessibility of out-of-hospital birth options. These factors contributed to Reena's experience in a system that she may not have been very familiar with but had to take part in for the birth of her child. This could have been be Reena's first experience in a hospital for a long stay. This might be one of many experiences that she'd had in a hospital. But one thing is for sure. The power of the hospital was very present because of factors that were mostly out of Reena's control. A lack of control equates to a lack of power, and a power imbalance can be abused by the person or entity in power.

We should also think about other power dynamics that were present in the birth experience for Reena. For example, Hilary, Reena's mother, definitely was the more powerful one in her interaction with Reena during the birth experience. She was Reena's elder, has had the experience of birthing multiple children, and just generally had more life experience that she constantly reminded Reena of. Then of course there was the mother-daughter dynamic and the automatic respect that comes with the label of being a mother, especially in Black culture where a child's opposing opinion can potentially be seen as disrespect.

For Jarrod there were also many power systems at play in his experience. If you think about it, one of his biggest fears was having an involuntary interaction with the criminal justice system. If he were to get too upset about the mistreatment or lack of attention to Reena, would he be deemed as dangerous and possibly be removed from the hospital, leaving Reena without his physical support? His experience as a Black man and the experience of other Black men in the South taught him to keep his head low because the criminal justice system was never there to protect him but to keep others protected from him. His reaction to even the thought of interacting with the criminal justice system left him in freeze and left him unable to be present in the ways that he wanted to, which would have included being more vocal and mentally present and less fearful during the birth of his child.

Samantha, the registered nurse, had some power in this interaction. She was one of the experts in this space as a labor and delivery registered nurse. She had also been working within this hospital system for some years and had gained lots of experiences from interacting with many different patients during their childbirth experiences. However, she also had some power struggles with the physician even though they both were in the medical system, as experts and as employees who were voluntarily part of the system. The physician had more power than Samantha. The physician had the power to say yes or no and to give Samantha a hard time if she did not agree with what he was putting forward. He could ultimately have Samantha removed as an employee if he felt it was necessary. That system of power pushed Samantha into not voicing as many concerns as she could have, which might have saved Reena's life, and instead pushed her into being subservient. Samantha was put in a position of choosing her own job safety over the health of the patient she was serving, which should never be a choice anyone has to make.

Dr. Smith seemed to hold the most power in this interaction. He had been a physician for years, with a plethora of experience. His position and power, as well as his external identities as a non-BIPOC cisgender male, created an image of power not many would question. He was aware of this truth as well, but internally he did not feel as powerful as most assumed. Although he was a physician, he was still under the influence of the hospital system and its policies, which he did not always agree with. However, after his negative experience going against hospital policy in the past and feeling the effects of that experience, he committed to letting the hospital system direct the way he cared for his patients, even if it meant going against his own knowledge and intuition. Dr. Smith often felt pressured to follow the one-size-fits-all ways of the health care system and was fearful of his reputation being negatively affected or even his medical license being suspended if he ever resisted any hospital practices or policy.

In the case of Reena, he thought about different ways to go about respecting Reena's goals and having a positive outcome, but he felt his hands were tied.

Questions that you may want to ask when analyzing power systems are:

- What power systems are currently in play?
- What power systems am I or my client interacting in, voluntarily and involuntarily?
- What are the effects of these power systems?
- How are the power systems making me feel emotionally, physically, semantically, and so on?
- Do I have the ability to choose how much or how little I interact with these power systems?
- Are there alternatives to this power system?
- How can I best support myself or others through an interaction with this power system?
- How do we best prepare ourselves to interact with the present power system?
- What are the experiences of people of certain identities, such as BIPOC people, in this power system?

Address Intersecting Oppressions

Intersectionality is the layered approach to examining the various identities of an individual or group (such as race, class, gender, body size, physical location, and education level) and understanding the interconnection of privileges or barriers experienced because of these identities.

Intersectionality was developed by Kimberlé Williams Crenshaw, a lawyer and civil rights and critical race theory advocate. The theory of intersectionality was created as a response to feminism centering whiteness, as well as ignoring issues such as sexuality, class, race, immigration, and ableism.

One of my favorite ways to talk about intersectionality is using the intersectionality wheel. If you search online, there are many interpretations of this wheel, but they all share the same idea. When looking at this wheel, you will notice that the middle of the wheel has the word *power*. And as you move farther out into the different layers of the wheel, you get more into marginalized identities. For example, in the section of the intersectionality wheel closest to power, you will find identities such as rich, English-speaking, cisgender man, post-secondary education, able-bodied, heterosexual, neurotypical, slim, and so on. These identities are usually most valued and prioritized in dominant culture, especially in the United States.

As you move to the second layer of the wheel, you will start to see identities such as middle class, speaking some English, different shades of skin color, high school education, some disability, some neurodivergence, average body size, and sheltered or renting. These identities are in the middle category of power. These identities are definitely not the center of power, but also aren't necessarily the most marginalized. The third and outermost layer of intersectionality wheel shows some of the most marginalized identities such as poor, non-English monolingual, dark skin color, significant disability, LGBTQIA+, vulnerable mental health, large body size, and homeless.

Why is this wheel important? I want you to look at this wheel and see how close or how far you are to power. I also want you to notice the ways in which your proximity to power is layered in this intersectionality wheel. In some ways you might be in a most marginalized layer, and in other ways you may be somewhere in between the first and second layer of the wheel. For example, I myself am a Black, dark-skinned, queer, average-sized, nonbinary woman, an American citizen, and middle class with mostly stable mental health. In that description of myself, I see ways that I fit within the most marginalized

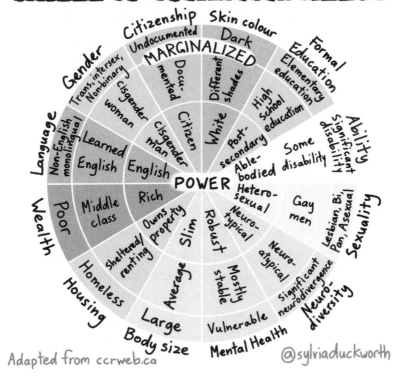

WHEEL OF POWER/PRIVILEGE

Citizenship   Skin colour

Gender   Undocumented   Dark

MARGINALIZED

Trans, intersex, Nonbinary   Documented   Different shades   Formal Education   Elementary education

cisgender woman   Citizen   White   High School   Post-secondary education

Language   cisgender man   English   Able-bodied   Some disability   Ability   Significant disability

Learned English   English   POWER   Hetero-sexual   Gay men

Non-English monolingual   Rich   Heterosexual   Gay men

Middle class   Slim   Robust   Neuro-typical   Lesbian, Bi, Pan, Asexual   Sexuality

Wealth   Poor   Owns property   Neuro-atypical

Sheltered/renting   Average   Mostly stable   Significant neurodivergence   Neuro-diversity

Homeless   Vulnerable   Mental Health

Housing   Large   Body size   Mental Health

Adapted from ccrweb.ca   @sylviaduckworth

identities as well as identities that put me closer to power. I do have some power in some ways—and in other spaces I do not. One of the important parts about intersectionality is that we are all very layered. It's so interesting that my identity as a Black, queer, nonbinary woman is something that I celebrate loudly and proudly. However, when I look at the way that dominant culture perceives me and even looking at this wheel, I realize the ways in which dominant culture may view my strengths as weaknesses and count me out, not taking me seriously during my pursuits in health, business, and so on.

Reena was twenty-six years old, Black, a heterosexual cisgender woman, college educated, middle class, neurotypical, and of average size. She was in ideal health by the standards of Western medicine. Her mother, Hilary, was a Black heterosexual cisgender woman, and middle aged, college educated, and had had a traumatic childbirth experience in a hospital. Jarrod was a Black cis male, high school educated and fearful of the criminal justice system. Samantha, the nurse, was a non-BIPOC cisgender woman, had experienced poverty, and was a single parent from Massachusetts. Dr. Smith was a non-BIPOC cisgender male physician from Virginia who had experienced a privileged life but had unresolved trauma from a prior childbirth experience with a patient.

You may notice that even using those identifiers and looking at the intersectionality wheel, some people had more power than others. Dr. Smith was a non-BIPOC citizen with many levels of postsecondary education. He was fairly well off financially because of his position, owned property, and didn't have many issues getting what he desired in life partially because of the many identities he held that are closer to power. Samantha also had many identifiers that put her in the power wheel, but also some that didn't, such as experiencing poverty. Being a single parent and being a cisgender woman are all things that move her away from the power center of dominant culture. Then you have Jarrod, a Black cisgender male. Being a male generally increases power, but when faced with structures in dominant culture, being a Black cis male decreases a person's power and his ability to be safe in public, as witnessed by the amount of Black cis men who are incarcerated and/or affected by police violence. Knowledge is power, so Jarrod being high school educated affected his ability to have more power. He had never had children and had never had any experience with the process of childbirth.

One of the important questions to ask ourselves when addressing intersecting opinions is: In what ways does this person notice how those identifiers created their experience? Also, remember to see experience as a power identifier—for example with Hilary, who had some identifiers that made her marginalized but also some that maybe enriched her experience, like being college educated and middle

REPRODUCTIVE JUSTICE . . . TO COLLECTIVE LIBERATION   79

class. Then there's Reena, who had some identifiers that marginalize her, such as being a Black cis woman. But she was also in ideal health for Western medicine standards and college educated—identities of privilege. When we consider these layers of being a Black woman interacting with the power system of the medical-industrial complex, we know statistically that the chance of her dying during childbirth, as well as the chance of her child dying within the first year of birth, greatly increase. The thing to notice is that each of these characters had things that can pull them toward the power center of dominant culture, as well as things that can push them further away from power.

Let's use the wheel to examine how power affects someone's interaction with the criminal justice system, focusing on Jarrod. If we were to seek an understanding of his fear of the criminal justice system, we might note, looking at this wheel, that he was a cis man, has a high school education, and is also Black. A white cis male interacting with the criminal justice system may not have as much fear or apprehension or experience with the criminal justice system because of the ways that he is closer to power and the ways statistics show he is not as likely to have a negative interaction with the criminal justice system. So again, when we're talking about intersecting oppressions, we're talking about getting a full picture, as full of a picture as we can possibly get for a view into the person's experience of life.

Although this wheel can be used to assist in narrowing down our identities and our relationship to power, we are more than even these categories. Using the power wheel as a tool of analysis and understanding can assist us in getting more perspective and asking more of the right questions, but it does not remove the nuance of power and identities. None of us are monoliths, so it is important to use these tools in conjunction with holding space for the information we may not see or learn, immediately or ever. If we only take in one or two identifiers, or we only focus on what we can see, then we miss out on perspective. We miss out on education. We miss out on the ability to provide trauma-informed care. We miss out on life-saving knowledge. We miss out on our ability to recognize our own bias and our own discrimination, which means we miss out on the ability to do something about it. Missing out on the ability to consciously do better and be better can be the end of a life like Reena's.

Questions you may ask yourself while evaluating for reproductive justice:

- What identities are currently present?
- Which identities are obvious?
- Which identities are not currently obvious but present?
- Do I need to know these identities, or can I move forward using trauma-informed principles without knowing the exact identities?
- How do I best address these intersecting identities?
- What identities am I familiar and comfortable with?
- What identities am I not familiar or comfortable with?
- Do I need to learn additional information or invest in further education because of these identities?
- Will I or others be doing a disservice to this client by serving them without much knowledge of these intersecting oppressions?
- Am I the best fit for this interaction, or is there a better fit or better resource for these intersecting identities?
- What is needed right now? What is not needed?
- How might my identities be affecting this experience? How do I acknowledge the benefits or drawbacks of my identities being present along with the identities presently served?

Center the Most Marginalized

When we think about the idea of collective liberation, it can feel like a big ask, and it can feel like an impossible mission, if I'm being honest. Collective liberation requires us to decenter ourselves and push forward with the mission of equity for all. When we think about centering the most marginalized, the truth that is present but not spoken about openly enough is that in order to do this, we must drop our egos and decenter ourselves and our experiences many times, understanding that if we can solve an issue for the most marginalized, then we can solve an issue for everyone. This can be hard work, especially when your identities are marginalized, especially when isms such as racism, ableism, and sexism create difficulties and barriers in your life because of your identities. This is even harder work if you aren't affected by the issue and you are being asked to put your energy into something you may not receive instant gratification from—or even a personal thank you. When it comes to the perinatal mortality rates, many people of all races and identities feel far removed from the problem and the solution, especially if they do not have children or aren't in a place to even fathom themselves as becoming parents. However, when we lose a friend or family member during childbirth or hear about someone close to us experiencing a loss related to birth, we suddenly feel pulled into this issue. What if instead, before tragedy struck or before we were closely connected to becoming a parent, we contributed to finding solutions to the Black birth disparities, understanding that if we could solve the most urgent and pressing matter for Black birthing people, we could also solve the smaller but still urgent matters of all birthing people? Our friends, family, and, most important, we ourselves could experience the process of being pregnant and going through childbirth with more safety, more knowledge, and an improved chance of survival, all because centering and solving the issues of the most marginalized has created more solutions for all. This practice of centering the most marginalized in order to improve other inequities and disparities can also be true for all people, including people who are in different phases of life, including nonpregnant people facing other health issues outside of the reproductive health scope. It is human nature to want to push forward on the things that affect us directly, and it is also human nature to want to avoid and ignore issues that do not directly impact us. But collective liberation is purposeful, which requires us to purposely act differently in order to reach the goal we are hoping to achieve: equity for all. My questions to you are: What if an issue doesn't affect you directly? Could you still center the most marginalized and put in work to assist in creating equity for the most marginalized? Could you put your ego aside, understanding that if we center the most marginalized, all of us will win? This desperate need for centering the most marginalized couldn't be any clearer than in our current disparities for Black birthing people and Black infants.

If you are a non-BIPOC person, I want you to be honest with yourself and your community. In those spaces it is important to discuss the requirements of being a white accomplice—pushing your ego aside in order to put your power toward the ongoing effort to assist BIPOC communities while also being directed by the BIPOC community. That would mean that we (BIPOC and non-BIPOC communities) will have to collectively join forces to push for safety, equity, and quality care for Black people. That also means that we will have to look beyond the labels that we carry—some of which sometimes pit us against each other—labels that go beyond race. For example, I've always been highly bothered by the separation of the in-hospital birth environment and the out-of-hospital birth environment. In some spaces just the mention of hospital-based certified nurse midwives and home-birth midwives causes a great deal of tension immediately. I often wonder, if we are all on the same mission to increase the quality of life for Black birthing people and their children, why can't we get beyond the ways that we are different? Obviously, there's many reasons for that. There's ego, history, legality, and there's just old-fashioned pent-up anger, which are all very valid. However, allowing that past history and maybe even current anger to keep us separated, unable to collaborate, unable to share experiences, and unable to share critical knowledge that could be literally lifesaving is one of the biggest failures of the birth world. What would it look like if across interdisciplinary positions, races, locations, and other factors we all decided to put our energy, time, or knowledge into creating accessible evidence based on lifesaving measures for Black birthing people and Black birthing infants?

In the case of Reena, we saw the breakdown of care due to not centering the most marginalized. Her life could have been saved if everyone would have gotten on the same page and centered her, the most marginalized (and vulnerable) in the space at the time. If questions were directed to her, if curiosity was directed to her, and if listening ears were directed to her, this experience could have been completely different. We must also trust that the most marginalized know themselves and that we are not the experts on their bodies. We must break the Western ideology of thinking that health is one size fits all. If we're going to center the most marginalized, we must listen to the most marginalized. We must take direction from the most marginalized. We must follow the most marginalized, understanding that life experience makes them the expert. That also means that even as professionals, whether we are doulas, doctors, lactation consultants, therapists, or holders of any other professional title, we must also understand that centering the most marginalized means sharing the power. It means giving back and returning the power that rightfully belongs to the affected person. In giving a person's power back to them in these power systems that we are all a part of, we most likely will have to go off route from these one-size-fits-all models of care and into more personalized and patient-centered approaches of care. That is the work.

The beautiful part about centering the most marginalized is that when we do so, and we solve and resolve issues that are present, such as racism and discrimination against Black people in the health care system, we then will know how to solve even more issues for other groups. If we can solve the hardest issue, then we can now spread this knowledge, with understanding of the factors that need to be personalized and led by the members of that group. If we can create ways to keep Black birthing people alive even through the most traumatic experiences, imagine the hope it will give others who are not as marginalized and who can greatly benefit from this knowledge and innovation. Medical technologies have been created to lessen health disparities, but they have not been able to decrease the specific issues that face Black birthing parents and infants. But if we can work together and learn how to keep more Black infants alive, well, and healthy beyond their first year of life, imagine the impact that we will have going forward for everyone. One of the scariest things that I realized after listening to Karen A. Scott, a Black feminist ob-gyn who has worked on Black perinatal health for over twenty years, was that 60 to 70 percent of the Black perinatal deaths happening are preventable. So that means that technology is not the problem. We have more than enough technology. We have the technology to decrease cesarean sections, to solve bacterial infections, and to even decrease the rates of postpartum hemorrhage. We have these things available to us, but still at the end of the day people are the ones who use this technology. We are the ones who decide whether and how it is to be used or not. We're talking about decreasing 60 to 70 percent of the deaths of Black perinatal birthing people. If we can solve the issue of explicit and implicit bias, which means creating systems of accountability, impact, and learning as well as systems of removing, then we can solve even more issues for everyone else who interacts with the birth roles.*

Questions to ask yourself:
- Who is currently the most marginalized in this interaction?
- What can I do to support the most marginalized person in this interaction?

---

* Karen Scott, "Black Mothers Matter: Racism and Childbirth in America," BBM Panel, *Hollywood Health and Society*, May 21, 2019, audio, 38:56, https://youtu.be /DVi46ErwY00.

- Am I centering myself, my pain, and/or my own trauma at the expense of actually creating rebirth of justice and collective liberation?
- Am I truly willing to share power in order to give power to marginalized communities?
- Do I struggle with censoring myself and my ego, and what can I do when these feelings come up?
- If I feel like I'm not equipped at the moment, what can I do to embody centering the most marginalized?
- What can I do to remove myself from the situation?
- What does it mean for me to be a white accomplice? What does it look like?

Join Together Across Issues and Identities

As I've continued to do this work of being a full-spectrum doula and reproductive justice advocate, as well as working through my own personal trauma and experiences, I have become very much aware of how colonization has created a part of me that always wants to feel important. The messaging I received through my life was the more I aligned with whiteness and colonization in my appearance and behavior, the more important and valuable my Black body became. An example of this is my desire to conquer versus collaborate. Much of our American history is about non-BIPOC communities creating value for themselves through the action of conquering rather than finding strength in collaborating and finding a healthy and agreed-upon way to coexist between communities. I found myself wanting to conquer, especially in work spaces, because I felt that if I didn't conquer, I would be deprioritized instead. Feeling important can look different ways for me. Sometimes I want to feel that whatever issue I'm going through is going to be the main issue or the main focus. Other times I just want people to know my identity, and celebrate and truly hear me and see nothing wrong with any of my feelings, whether they be anger, happiness, joy, jealousy, or complete exhaustion. However, when it comes to this work of collective liberation, it is important to recognize the spaces in ourselves that aim for destructive separation from others. What I mean by that is we all tend to miss opportunities, especially in the movements for justice like Black Lives Matter and Trans Lives Matter. There's no doubt that all these movements matter and need funding and support to get their initiatives moving forward constantly and consistently. There is power in numbers, and when they are separated they tend to lose their power because of the smaller amounts of accumulated power, money, support, and more. However, when many organizations came together during the 2020 protests under the one mission of Black lives being valued, mountains moved and highly privileged communities were forced to pay attention because of the fear of the numbers produced at these protests and the unity across all races, genders, and peoples for this vital movement.

Joining together across issues and identities creates power and strength in numbers by building a solid force of humans in a similar mindset, generating resources and building consistency (a.k.a. staying ready so we don't have to get ready!). In my organization, Birthing Advocacy Doula Trainings (BADT), I have strived to create a space where everyone can be seen and heard and remain important—but also can gather across issues and identities. The more we gather, the more impact we can have. This was especially on display in 2020 during the racial uprisings after the murders of George Floyd, Ahmaud Arbery, and Breonna Taylor. I am so proud to say BADT members with many different identities went into action, providing mutual aid, being present at protests, being street medics, and finding many other ways they could support Black community members. There was a mutual understanding that protecting Black community members was the mission, and it did not mean other issues weren't important; it just meant that this was the most urgent and that it deserved as much collective time, energy, and resources that we could put toward the issue as possible.

There's also beauty in the fact that when we gather, we can then take information that we have learned separately and bring it together for the goal of collective liberation. The benefit of gathering and sharing information is that I don't have to learn all aspects to make this change happen. Perhaps I know two of the things, and you know three of the things, and this other group knows four other things, and so on, so when we come together, we now have a full picture, a fuller perspective, and the fullest force. I am human also, so I know that it can be hard to hold space and focus on a cause that isn't affecting you as intensely as it faces the most marginalized while you are personally being completely affected by another issue that is impacting your security and your identity, and that is pushing you to the edge mentally, spiritually, physically, and emotionally. I don't believe in utopias, but I believe in your ability to work toward collective liberation, which will require patience, self-regulation, consistency, and anger. We can and should put full force into the most marginalized communities and help to solve a problem or to make an impact. Then we move to another community that is most marginalized and also needs the full force of the collective to share information, put plans into action, and make an impact in a timely and efficient manner.

When I look at the things that have happened and the different movements in the last few years (LGBTQIA+ rights, #MeToo, Black Lives Matter, marijuana legalization and decriminalization, Indigenous rights, etc.), I see a pattern that when people of different identities and espousing different issues come together, things seem to be addressed faster. Legislation has evolved, and culture has shifted greatly. Advocates are presented with options faster, and at times come to solutions that are helpful or at least a step forward. I want to emphasize that this is where it's *very* important for white accomplices to be physically, mentally, and financially present for these causes. Black Lives Matter was created in 2013. Through those initial years, BLM gained traction, became well known, especially in organizing spaces, and also dealt with a large amount of backlash from many communities. Then continuous and highly publicized murders of unarmed Black people took place in 2020, including the murders of Breonna Taylor and George Floyd. As these murders were happening, the coronavirus pandemic was in its early stages and starting to affect not only BIPOC communities but non-BIPOC communities as well. The mix of these factors created a time when non-BIPOC people were the most present I have ever seen in my life. Non-BIPOC communities were consistently present at Black Lives Matter protests, as well as active in the pandemic relief protests as well. All of a sudden, pandemic relief checks were hitting accounts, companies were issuing statements in support of Black Lives Matter, and even police were being fired and/or arrested for their crimes. I remember feeling like I was in some alternate world, and I realized that change was happening fast because non-BIPOC people with power and privilege were present in building a force I had never truly seen before in my life. During these protests, abuses of force from the police became a regular factor. As a result of that, many non-BIPOC protesters decided to use their bodies to circle and protect BIPOC protesters from violence, and in many cases, this worked. These protesters were white accomplices who truly understood their ability to use their bodies as a shield of safety for BIPOC communities, understanding that the chance of their bodies being devalued and harmed was minimal compared to BIPOC individuals.

That is the power of being a non-BIPOC person in the United States—that even through chaos, violence, and uncertainty, there is still a level of privilege and physical safety present at all times. That is the reason why non-BIPOC people must join with BIPOC folks across the issues that affect BIPOC communities. That is how non-BIPOC people yield their power and do the actual work of being a white accomplice led by the BIPOC community.

I have also noticed that in the United States, there is a conscious and subconscious desire for us to feel important and be at the top of the hierarchical systems we all take part in, whether it's our income level, education level, or amount of experience in a specific topic. These hierarchical systems distract us from moving forward because we are too focused on who's better. We push the lived experiences of marginalized communities out of the conversation instead of focusing on what issues matter most and which individuals or groups are truly best to lead the movement toward sustainable and long-term solutions and change.

For example, we see the level of importance being played out in the government by such things as funding. In 2019 my nonprofit, For the Village, began a long-term collaboration with another organization that we love. One of the first things that I learned moving into that collaboration—which was told to me in an apologetic way—was now that our collaborator had changed their direction to focus on Black birthing people, the budgets had been cut. However, the aim was still to serve nearly as many birthing people that were served in the previous years before funding was decreased. I remember thinking about that disconnect and having to make a decision to move forward even with these deficits being present. Even though statistically these power systems (medical-industrial complex, government, nonprofit organizations, etc.) knew the most marginalized are Black birthing people, and we see it plastered all over pamphlets and such, there was (and still is) this inequity in how much funding would be available for the issue that we know is the most urgent and in crisis at this time.

With all that said, I also understood that impactful change, encompassing in its entirety all the above elements, requires more than just money. It requires people on the same page and ready to do the work utilizing their different identities, knowledge, privileges, and access points. Can you imagine if non-BIPOC people put in this type of anger, consistency, and protection of BIPOC communities into the disparities currently affecting Black birth people and our children? What change could be made? What initiatives could be funded and able to push forward? The force of the collective creates change.

Questions you may ask yourself to assist in moving into sustainable action:

- How are you truly willing to show up?
- Are you willing to take a look at what issues are an emergency and put work into them even if they aren't directly connected to your experience?
- Would you be able to accept that causes that do affect you will be worked on but may be worked on consistently and possibly at a slower pace?
- Are you willing to do the work of self-regulation and joining together with people who may not always agree with you in every way for the goal of collective liberation?
- If I'm seeking collective liberation, who am I willing to join for that mission to happen?
- What are my boundaries across interacting with specific issues or specific identities?
- How will I deal with the discomfort that may come with working closely with people who may have both aligned and unaligned thoughts?

5

UNPACKING TRAUMA AS A PERSONAL RESPONSIBILITY

Fire can warm or consume,
water can quench or drown,
wind can caress or cut.
And so it is with human relationships:
we can both create and destroy,
nurture and terrorize,
traumatize and heal each other.

—Bruce Perry, *The Boy Who Was Raised as a Dog*

TRAUMA CAN BE defined in many different ways. The American Psychological Association defines trauma as "an emotional response to a terrible event like an accident, rape, or natural disaster." *Merriam-Webster* defines trauma as "a disordered psychic or behavioral state resulting from severe mental or emotional stress or physical injury, or an emotional upset."* All great definitions—but I have chosen to define trauma as an event or change that someone *personally* registers as too much, too fast, too soon. I specifically have used the word *personally* in the definition because only the individual can determine if or when something feels traumatic. For example, I attended a birth with a client who was being induced for medical reasons, and she was given Pitocin (a synthetic form of oxytocin, used to induce labor by increasing the strength and frequency of contractions) in the childbirth process. Within a couple hours, her contractions were strong and consistent, but in my opinion, it was too quick of a change in intensity and could be traumatic for the client. However, when I checked in with the client, she agreed about the intensity but felt excited about what was happening and looked forward to the chance to officially meet her child soon. In that experience, I had to practice my skill set of regulating myself and my own feelings in order to be present for my client and their feelings of being completely aligned and in agreement with the direction of their childbirth experience. In another experience, my clients have shared parts of their pregnancy and childbirth experiences that I registered as routine and normal but that they felt traumatized by. In each and every experience I have with clients, or anyone, I have learned to trust what feels like too much, too fast, too soon in their personal interpretation and use this information to meet them where they are, without judgment or the pressure to

---

* Merriam-Webster, "Trauma," *Merriam-Webster*, accessed June 15, 2022, https://www.merriam-webster.com/dictionary/trauma.

prove that they did in fact experience trauma. It's also important to note that while someone's trauma can feel big or small to you, never measure trauma by size. Instead, accept it as a very present and real part of a person's lived experience, which is the only factor that matters.

Another important fact to note about trauma is that it is usually created with the assistance of an external factor that is out of our control. For example, after finally receiving the uterine fibroid diagnosis, I felt very traumatized by my experience of seeing multiple doctors and not receiving a proper diagnosis, even after doing all that I could to advocate for myself. I often thought about what would have happened if I hadn't seen the third doctor who referred me to get an MRI and caught the fibroid before it grew even larger. Could I have been severely affected or even died? I wasn't able to be in control of the actions of the doctors who dismissed me, and their dismissal could have been my demise. The lack of control fueled my anxiety, and months after those interactions, I was still feeling very angry and fearful of trusting my health care providers, especially because I was dealing with further complications stemming from the original uterine fibroid.

However, as time passed, I realized I didn't want to constantly feel the physical and mental manifestations of my health care trauma, and I decided to start taking steps to heal this part of myself. I did not create this trauma, but it was my personal responsibility to heal it, simply because no one else could do that work for me and I deserved to not carry the weight of that trauma on my shoulders from day to day. For me, healing that particular point of trauma included continuing to advocate for others through my work as a doula, attending therapy previously, doing things that nourished my body, and having people and rituals in my life that honored my pain, a place that had never known love. For you, healing your trauma may be through reading this book, being around people who pour into you, taking part in healing modalities, and ultimately realizing that although you did not create this trauma, it is your responsibility to heal it. It is not an easy responsibility, and honestly sometimes it feels like it isn't a fair responsibility to have. But it is what is needed and appreciated if we are truly aiming for collective liberation.

With trauma comes trauma responses. Responses to trauma can look completely different from individual to individual. One person experiencing trauma may sit quietly and very still, and may even look like they are "keeping it together." Another person may become angry and lash out verbally and physically, while another person may decide to leave the space or situation as soon as possible in order to relieve their negative feelings. All these reactions are normal, but some of these reactions are more socially accepted than others. Some reactions are more accepted by a particular set of individuals due to factors such as race. How many of us have seen a non-BIPOC male lash out verbally and not receive much, if any, consequence, but if a Black male has the same reaction, that can result in violence, jail time, and even death? This was the experience of Jarrod.

Somatic Exercise: What Does Trauma Mean to You?

Trauma, like many things in this human experience, isn't one size fits all, even if we only use this one word to describe an experience that can look completely different from person to person. In my experience, I have even had internal battles of deciding what counted as trauma in my life because I wanted to grade each experience as being big or small. Trauma can be an interaction that lasts days, hours, or even seconds. It can also be an interaction that may not have felt like a big deal to anyone else but yourself, and that is OK too. I believe it is important to get acquainted with trauma in a personal way by understanding what we define as trauma for ourselves, especially because the traumas that we may define as "small" are still affecting us in some way, so it's best to recognize the full spectrum of trauma we are working with and within in our personal lives.

Create a comfortable space for yourself, grab a paper and pen, and answer the following questions as honestly as you can without feeling shame over what may come to your mind. If answering these questions begins to feel overwhelming, you are welcome to pause and return or stop and move forward. Remember this book is meant to be a guide, and if permission is needed, I welcome you to participate in each exercise (or not), honoring the limits your body and mind are presenting to you.

1. When you think of trauma, what thoughts come to mind? How does your body react to these thoughts? Take notice if your thoughts are general thoughts about trauma or more personalized to your living experience.

2. Do you consider yourself to be someone who has experienced trauma? Are there any emotions, thoughts, or physical sensations that come up when asking yourself this question?

3. What does trauma feel like in your body, if there is any present? Physical sensations could be a heavy chest, tingling sensations, and/or a physical pain in a specific area of your body. Emotions such as numbness, anger, sadness, or even the desire to laugh can also come up to the surface.

4. What would it be like to give yourself full permission to heal? This is not to be confused with trauma being gone at the snap of a finger, but it does mean giving yourself the time, space, and care that you need in order to create an ongoing healing journey.

Spend time with these questions and allow yourself to feel into your response physically, just as much as you are thinking into your response.

Before we get deeper into the detail of the trauma responses, I'd like to give you a bit more foundational knowledge that will assist us in attaining a better understanding of the four trauma responses. All our bodies consist of a central nervous system that contains our brain (the central computer of our body) and our spinal cord (the connecting network of nerves that relay messages back and forth from the brain to parts of our bodies). Your brain and spinal cord make up the central nervous system (CNS), and the nerves that go through the entire body make up the peripheral nervous system (PNS). The autonomic nervous system (ANS) is a part of the peripheral nervous system and helps us survive. It houses the control center for things like how fast or deep we breathe, the muscle contractions of the heart, and blood pressure. The autonomic nervous system has two components, one being the sympathetic nervous system, and the other the parasympathetic nervous system. The sympathetic nervous system is what jumps into action when we experience a dangerous or stressful occurrence. The physical manifestation of the sympathetic nervous system in action usually looks like an adrenaline rush, breathing faster, making physical moves without always being conscious of them, or even running away. The parasympathetic system directs the body to calm down or to "rest and digest." This system can balance the sympathetic system by assisting the body into slow breathing, slow movement, and find its way back to homeostasis, or balance.

Again, I want to remind you that your responses to trauma are normal. The beautiful part about trauma responses is that they are our body's way of protecting us so we can move through and even survive the experience. There are four trauma responses: fight, flight, freeze, and fawn. I will define each trauma response, explain how they may look outwardly, and give an example from Reena's story. As we are working through these definitions and examples, I would also like for you to notice if you or anyone around you have exhibited these trauma responses. Think about how you might reframe your thoughts

PERIPHERAL AUTONOMIC NERVOUS SYSTEM

PARASYMPATHETIC   SYMPATHETIC

PUPIL CONSTRICTION   DILATED PUPILS

STIMULATE SALIVA   INHIBIT SALIVATION

NERVUS VAGUS

CONSTRICTS BRONCHI   RELAXES BRONCHI

SYMPATHETIC
TRUNK NODES   INCREASED
                                                      HEARTBEAT
SLOW HEART RATE
SOLAR PLEXUS
SYMPATHETIC   SLOWS
NERVE FIBERS   DOWN DIGESTION
SUPERIOR
STIMULATES   MESENTERIC   STIMULATES
PRODUCTION OF BILE   NODE   GLUCOSE RELEASE

STIMULATES   REDUCES
DIGESTION   INTESTINAL
                              INFERIOR   MUSCLES
                              MESENTERIC
                              NODE
INTESTINAL   ADRENALINE
MUSCLE   PRODUCTION
RELAXATION

SPINAL NERVES

CAUSES AN ERECTION   REDUCES BLOOD FLOW

MAINTAINS HOMEOSTASIS   MOBILIZES RESERVES
                                               UNDER STRESS

Macrovector/Shutterstock

around your own or others' responses by including compassion and understanding.

Fight is the desire to fight back, and it activates the parasympathetic nervous system. Reading the word *fight* can create assumptions about the fight response being a negative response to an experience, usually including physical combativeness or verbal assault. An unhealthy fight response can look like controlling behaviors, creating unnecessary conflict, narcissism, and even bullying. A healthy fight response can include being assertive, establishing and maintaining firm boundaries, and protecting yourself and others when necessary.

During Reena's childbirth, Hilary, her mother, displayed many examples of the fight trauma response. Some of those moments include comparing every aspect of her birth to Reena's experience, having a visceral reaction to Dr. Smith's C-section suggestion, and getting noticeably frustrated when Jarrod told her she needed to calm down. Nurse Samantha also experienced the fight response when Dr. Smith told her to schedule a C-section and she chose to speak up about her disagreement with his suggestion, even though questioning a doctor's opinion was against normal protocol. Upon being questioned, Dr. Smith went into his fight response by tensely explaining his suggestion and demonstrating his authority because he felt threatened by Samantha. What other instances in Reena's story stick out to you as a fight response?

Flight is the desire to leave the immediate area and happens when the parasympathetic nervous system takes a back seat. The flight response is usually activated when a person feels they cannot face what's in front of them (whether it be because of physical or emotional barriers), so their response is to leave the present situation completely. An unhealthy flight response can include avoidance of feeling tough feelings, needing to stay busy at all times, exhibiting obsessive or compulsive tendencies, experiencing constant panic and fear, or even desiring perfection. A healthy flight response can include assessing danger, removing yourself or others from a physically dangerous situation, leaving an unhealthy relationship, or disengaging from harmful conversations.

A good example of this is Hilary stating that she did not trust the hospital or care providers and then deciding to leave the room for some fresh air without an explanation when Reena needed her to be present. At that time, we can assume Hilary felt powerless toward the medical-industrial complex, and although her mistrust was present, she felt she had no choice but to interact with this system and went into the flight response in order to try to maintain homeostasis through her current experience. Another example of flight is the moment when Dr. Smith, after stating that he was able to save the baby but not Reena, briskly walked away instead of dealing with the inevitable feelings of anger, sadness, and despair that would be felt by Hilary and Jarrod. What other instances in Reena's story stick out to you as a flight response?

Freeze is the inability to respond, instead "playing dead"—a response that primarily activates the parasympathetic nervous system. An unhealthy freeze response can include isolation, the perception of laziness, fear of trying new things, brain fog, and dissociation. A healthy freeze response can include awareness, mindfulness, and the ability to be fully present in the moment.

Jarrod experienced freeze when he wanted to speak up for Reena and ask questions about the care she was receiving but instead became quiet and even numb as he navigated not wanting to cause any issues, knowing that his desire to take part in leading the experience could be perceived as an unhealthy fight response from the employees in the hospital. Another example of freeze is Reena's respond to Dr. Smith when he told her and her family to start thinking about a cesarean section as an option because she had been laboring for twenty-four hours. Reena maintained eye contact but couldn't give any further signs of her thoughts or questions because at that moment she felt stuck and began to disassociate. An emergency surgical procedure was not at all what she wanted to experience, but she felt she had no choice. What other instances in Reena's story stick out to you as a freeze response?

Fawn is the desire to gain approval using conflict-avoidant behaviors in an attempt to diffuse a situation. It primarily activates the parasympathetic nervous system. The fawn response is the least-known trauma response, but it is so helpful in understanding ourselves and others. Many people who experience the fawn response have been around negative or toxic people for long periods of time and have learned to ease the threat by going above and beyond the call. An unhealthy fawn response can include loss of self, people-pleasing at the risk of self, having little to no boundaries, and participating in codependent, sometimes violent, relationships. A healthy fawn response can include active listening, compromise, and compassion for others.

When Dr. Smith decided to give Reena a C-section, Nurse Samantha did not agree with his choice. As I mentioned previously, she decided to stand up to Dr. Smith and was met with his tense and authoritative feedback. Samantha's response to quickly shift her approach and tell him he knew best while following his direction to prep Reena for surgery was a fawn response. At that moment, Samantha felt her livelihood being threatened by Dr. Smith, and her fear of being homeless again quickly pushed her into people-pleasing behaviors to remain "good" in the doctor's eyes. What other instances in Reena's story stick out to you as a fawn response?

TRAUMA RESPONSES

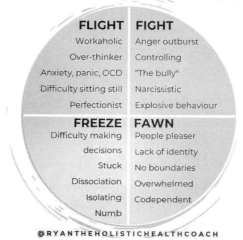

FLIGHT	FIGHT
Workaholic	Anger outburst
Over-thinker	Controlling
Anxiety, panic, OCD	"The bully"
Difficulty sitting still	Narcissistic
Perfectionist	Explosive behaviour

FREEZE	FAWN
Difficulty making decisions	People pleaser
	Lack of identity
Stuck	No boundaries
Dissociation	Overwhelmed
Isolating	Codependent
Numb	

@RYANTHEHOLISTICHEALTHCOACH

Racism as a Trauma

Through years of research, it has been proven time and again that racism and discrimination are the cause of past, current, and ongoing Black perinatal and infant mortality rates. I have been blessed to host many workshops and spaces where I talk about these topics, and as I began meeting more and more individuals of different races, cultures, and backgrounds, I realized that racism in itself is a trauma. Through the works of educators such as Resmaa Menakem, Rachel Cargle, Ibram X. Kendi, Britney Packnett Cunningham, and more, I have learned that racism is a trauma we are all experiencing, on an ongoing and regular basis. When I began to frame racism as a trauma in my personal and professional life, I started to listen to my students differently, and I was able to hear myself and others in a more expansive perspective.

In conversations about race, my students expressed feeling unable to talk, wanting to avoid the conversation, having angry outbursts, and wanting to do whatever they can to diffuse the conversation even at the sacrifice of themselves when talking about race. All examples of trauma responses. In many interactions with non-BIPOC people, white fragility was a frequent reaction. According to Robin DiAngelo, the author of *White Fragility,* the term refers to "the defensive reactions that white people have when [their] racial worldviews, positions, or advantages are questioned or challenged."[*] White fragility can include fear, fleeing a situation, anger, silence, and, of course, white tears. If we look beyond the visible responses and into the why, we can notice that these, too, are trauma responses.

Generally speaking, most of us can understand racism as a trauma for BIPOC folks. BIPOC folks are the victims of racism and for generations have dealt with the effects of racism, including disparities such as the wealth gap, high rates of incarceration, the school-to-prison

---

[*] Robin DiAngelo, "Ziet Campus Transcript," accessed June 15, 2022, https://robindiangelo .com/wp-content/uploads/2018/08/zeit-campus-transcript.pdf.

pipeline, and negative Black perinatal and infant mortality rates. We can also see the effects of racism-based trauma in the emotional and the physical states of BIPOC individuals, including higher rates of high blood pressure, diabetes, and other health outcomes, as well as trauma disorders and mental health disorders, such as depression and anxiety.

It can, however, be harder to understand the trauma effects on non-BIPOC people when it comes to racism. Reflecting back on non-BIPOC trauma responses to racism, I believe non-BIPOC people have these responses due to their lack of capacity for difference and change. For example, with outwardly racist non-BIPOC folks protesting against Black Lives Matter, I often notice that though these people may be externally showing anger and hatred, internally the root of this is fear: the fear of not being cared about, having to share power and space, and not being prioritized as much as they have previously been. That fear is the trauma that has been passed down through non-BIPOC generations that have experienced feeling important and validated through stealing resources, enslaving other humans, and being feared by BIPOC communities. As the tides are slowly shifting, the reaction has been to hold on to these prior ways of living as tightly as possible, and the more fear that is experienced, the more acting out we see. Some of that acting out has been seen in protests and even larger events, such as the January 6 Insurrection.

I would also like to mention that historically, BIPOC communities have always had to adjust to non-BIPOC communities, whether it has been regulating our attitudes, the way we dress, or the way we speak—but now non-BIPOC people are having to learn to adjust to BIPOC communities, which has also created these trauma responses for non-BIPOC people as they are forced to change. For example, as BIPOC people continue to find themselves in spaces we did not have access to before, especially leadership positions, non-BIPOC people are now learning to adjust to seeing BIPOC people in control of spaces and expanding access to other BIPOC folks to enter these spaces. In the last couple years, I have been able to build successful businesses and make connections with many different people who have invited me into spaces that are majority, if not completely, non-BIPOC spaces. Many people have asked me how I deal with this pressure and discomfort at times. Do I switch the way I talk or make any adjustments to create more safety for the non-BIPOC people in the space? My answer is always no. Because I recognize the lack of capacity for difference and change that haunts non-BIPOC people, I have purposely decided to be as close to myself as possible in hopes of that exposure creating a positive experience that can be a starting or continuing space for their healing.

> *Our bodies have a form of knowledge that is different from our cognitive brains. This knowledge is typically experienced as a felt sense of constriction or expansion, pain or ease, energy or numbness. Often this knowledge is stored in our bodies as wordless stories about what is safe and what is dangerous. The body is where we fear, hope, and react; where we constrict and release; and where we reflexively fight, flee, or freeze. If we are to upend the status quo of white-body supremacy, we must begin with our bodies.*
>
> —Resmaa Menakem, *My Grandmother's Hands: Racialized Trauma and the Pathway to Mending Our Hearts and Bodies**

The ultimate truth is that collective liberation requires ongoing collective healing. My healing is your healing. The healing of BIPOC and non-BIPOC communities and the trauma of racism is interconnected

---

* Resmaa Menakem, *My Grandmother's Hands: Racialized Trauma and the Pathway to Mending Our Hearts and Bodies* (Las Vegas: Central Recovery Press, 2017), chapter 1.

and impossible without the other. We are all inhabiting this world together. Even if we may not directly be in contact with one another, we are dependent on each other in many ways, from the emotional dependence we have on each other in our close relationships to the more logistical independence we share, such as getting care from a doctor or for necessities like food and water. Many of us tend to focus our healing on our individual selves, which is totally fine, but then when we walk out into the world and deal with people who are suffering and not on a healing journey, we quickly notice how much their trauma affects our lives as well. The next step to our individual healing process is to begin to call in others; those others may not be like you or even easy to talk to, but if we are going to get to this space of collective liberation and ongoing collective healing, this is the work we all must do.

Forms of Racism

Before we dive into some of the more detailed parts of trauma, I believe it is important to understand the forms of racism that contribute to race-based trauma. Many people tend to think about the obvious (or explicit) examples of racism, such as calling a BIPOC person a derogatory name or events such as the many unprovoked killings of BIPOC individuals by police officers. There are also more hidden and subconscious (or implicit) forms of racism occurring around us every day, like professional dress codes that discourage Black people from wearing their hair in its natural state or the repeated mispronunciation of an Indigenous name because it is "too hard" to say an Indigenous name correctly. Explicit and implicit bias contribute to race-based stress, and so do different forms of racism we may not always be aware of because they are happening on a systemic level, not just individual or interpersonal. Trauma comes from not just a person-to-person interaction but also from a system-to-person interaction. Understanding different forms of racism can assist with giving a better and fuller understanding of race-based trauma and can allow us to create more clarity around ways to dismantle racism and create a new and liberated world.

Individual Racism

Individual racism can be seen when one person holds particular beliefs or prejudices (either conscious or subconscious) about someone of a particular race that are purely based on stereotypes. Individual racism is obvious in people who have chosen to be openly racist by sharing their closed-minded and harmful thoughts about BIPOC people. It can also be displayed covertly and subconsciously through an individual implicit bias. The US Department of Health has indicated that, based on a set of quality measures and standards, Black and Latinx people are 40 percent less likely to receive quality care. This statistic speaks to the long-term effects of individual racism.* An example of this is an ob-gyn with a stellar reputation treating two clients, one Black and the other non-BIPOC, with the same exact medical conditions. The ob-gyn sends the non-BIPOC patient for further testing, gives them a narcotic pain medication, and schedules a follow-up in one week. However, the ob-gyn sends the Black patient home with ibuprofen and a note to get off work for a couple days in order to rest, and then schedules a follow-up visit in six weeks.

In this case, the ob-gyn does not have a conscious awareness of their racism, and this lack of awareness has influenced their decision to provide fewer resources for the Black patient and treat their follow-up appointment with less urgency. The ob-gyn did not mean to cause any intentional harm, but the unconscious individual racist thoughts influenced the lack of care provided to the Black patient in

---

* "Executive Summary," 2019 National Healthcare Quality and Disparities Report, AHRQ, December 2020, 7, https://www.ahrq.gov/sites/default/files/wysiwyg/research/findings/nhqrdr/2019qdr.pdf.

a way that can lead to further complications and even death if they are not treated with the same urgency and care as the non-BIPOC patient (implicit bias). Implicit bias occurs when an individual holds subconscious assumptions about people based on stereotypes.

On the flip side, this situation could also be true of an ob-gyn who makes these same choices based on their conscious individual racist thoughts (explicit bias). Explicit bias occurs when an individual holds assumptions often based on stereotypes, but this time they are conscious of their beliefs and attitudes toward a particular group of people.

Interpersonal Racism

Interpersonal racism is clear and evident racism occurring between individuals. Anarcha, the Black enslaved woman tortured with thirty surgeries without anesthesia by James Marion Sims, was a victim of interpersonal racism. Sims held explicit racist thoughts of Anarcha being inferior because of her race that therefore influenced his interpersonal racist actions of maintaining her enslavement, brutalizing her body with surgical procedures without anesthesia, and feeling justified in his purpose of finding a solution to a medical condition through violence against enslaved women. In present-day times, interpersonal racism is happening all around us, and it goes beyond name-calling and physical fights between racial groups. Recent examples of interpersonal racism include the death of Breonna Taylor, as well as the death of Amber Rose Isaac, a Black mother who died during childbirth less than four days after tweeting that she should write an exposé on "dealing with incompetent doctors." When explicit and implicit individual racist thoughts influence racist actions between two or more individuals, interpersonal racism is taking place. It is also important to note that even well-meaning interactions between BIPOC and non-BIPOC people can produce interpersonal racism, and non-BIPOC people should not get hung up on the idea of being racist but instead accept that racism has been programmed into our daily existence—so they must move beyond the label and focus on a plan of corrective action instead.

Cultural Racism

Cultural racism is the practice of broadcasting standards as the norm in a society, effectively defining something as the accepted culture. When thinking about standards of beauty or even standards of professionalism, usually non-BIPOC people are used as the prototype, even if these standards are derisive to BIPOC communities. For example, as a Black person navigating professional spaces, I often was told that professionalism meant mimicking non-BIPOC culture, especially when it came to my hair. I was much more palatable when my hair was relaxed, straight, and closer to the texture of a non-BIPOC person's hair. When I began to become more acquainted with who I am in my natural state, I decided to wear my hair in braids. These braids were neatly done and, in my opinion, beautiful, but I soon noticed the looks I received at work—and those looks later became negative feedback about my "professionalism." Nothing had changed about me except my appearance.

Cultural racism also takes place in the birth room in instances such as a nurse not respecting the traditional cultural needs of a Latinx birthing person because the nurse feels it is "weird" or unnecessary. Cultural racism requires BIPOC people to conform to non-BIPOC standards, sometimes for safety, or be left to deal with the consequences of choosing not to conform. I, personally, have left many positions in corporate America for exactly this reason. BIPOC people should not have to choose between their livelihood and their well-being, but this is the decision many BIPOC people come across when they decide not to conform in respect to themselves, their ancestors, and the future of BIPOC communities that will have to inhabit these spaces.

Institutional Racism

Institutional racism occurs when an institution, organization, or company has particular policies or practices in place that negatively impact a particular racial group while, as a result, helping another. A great example of this is the lack of diverse imagery currently available to birth professionals, such as physicians and nurses, in practice and in school. As I was building my doula career, I didn't notice at first how infrequently I saw images similar to myself in the visual resources I was consuming. Luckily, while searching for imagery for my organization, Birthing Advocacy Doula Trainings, I came across a resource called The Educated Birth (TEB), where founder Cheyenne Varner creates and curates inclusive reproductive health education and storytelling content. TEB blew my mind with all its illustrations, from diagrams of infants in utero to the images of lactation and pregnancy, that include all races, genders, physical abilities, and other diverse identities. I also realized that the lack of representation in educational resources in institutional settings, such as medical schools and hospitals, has been a choice that harms people of color in ways such as leaving medical professionals inexperienced with how BIPOC people may look physically during a reproductive health experience or complication, and that this lack of knowledge could be the difference between a BIPOC patient getting the correct care needed and not. More important, lack of representation in these spaces has been a choice made by these institutions because these resources exist but are not being utilized.

Another example of institutional racism is the field of research. Many of the standards we use today are based on a small group of research participants who usually did not include BIPOC people. Currently, BMI (body mass index) is a tool used by health care systems to determine the health of a person based on the amount of fat on their body compared to their height. This index was created by Adolphe Quetelet (who did not study medicine, by the way, and never intended his tool to be used as an indicator of individual health), and he created the BMI formula based on French and Scottish participants only, under the popular misconception that people of color were a subspecies. BMI was made for the use of understanding white European communities only, but it is still in use now for all people as a measure of an individual's health, and it increases harm to BIPOC people especially, as we were never meant to utilize this tool to begin with.* Even with this information, many institutions still rely on BMI and have not made revisions to decrease harm for BIPOC communities.

It's important to bring awareness to discussions of institutional racism that end with the institution saying they didn't consciously make a choice to be racist. In those times, I remind them that not making a choice by being negligent or being consciously or subconsciously exclusionary with a topic that is negatively affecting BIPOC communities is, in fact, still a choice.

Systemic (or Structural) Racism

Systemic (or structural) racism occurs when systems have laws or policies deeply submerged in the makeup and history that perpetuate harm toward a specific racially identified group. We've talked about a lack of BIPOC representation in health care, especially in positions that require higher education, and this is a form of systemic racism. There is disproportionate representation of women of color and immigrants in direct care positions, such as certified nursing assistants. According to Health Affairs, "certified nursing assistants' median yearly earnings in 2019 was $29,640, a rate that falls well below the median rate for women across all occupations ($41,028),

---

* Your Fat Friend, "The Bizarre and Racist History of the BMI," Elemental, October 15, 2019, https://elemental.medium.com/the-bizarre-and-racist-history-of-the-bmi -7d8dc2aa33bb.

and most nursing assistants remain low earners throughout their careers."* In institutions such as hospitals, there are policies that set the lowest and highest amount of salary each position can be offered. The low salaries of certified nursing assistants create an environment of low-wage workers, mostly BIPOC, who are unable to obtain a higher education in order to climb the career ladder because they are underpaid and often overworked without long-term support to provide them with the foundation to move into positions where they are needed in their communities. If policies in these institutions would change to mandate a higher wage, the power of BIPOC communities being affected by these low wages would increase by creating access to higher education and the ability to pursue higher-paying positions, as well as by allowing them to utilize their time to be more present for themselves and their families.

Knowing these forms of racism will allow each of us to understand the fullness of racism and its traumatic effects on all of us. Racism is not just a person. Racism can be a policy, a choice, a system, an institute, an action, or even a lack of action. Creating a fuller perspective of racism gives us the ability to understand how racism impacts us on a conscious and subconscious level and how it impedes our lives countless times throughout our day. The big difference is that depending on what side of racism we may be on, BIPOC or non-BIPOC, racism may look or feel different—but it is all trauma, regardless of whom the racism is directly impacting.

PTSD and CPTSD

We have dived into individual trauma, a trauma that occurs to a person individually, as well as racialized trauma, the traumatic response

---

* Janette Dill et al., "Addressing Systemic Racial Inequity in the Health Care Workforce," *Health Affairs*, September 10, 2020, https://www.healthaffairs.org/do/10.1377/forefront.20200908.133196.

to stress following a racial encounter. Post-traumatic stress disorder (PTSD) and complex post-traumatic stress disorder (CPTSD) are also very important to mention in this conversation of unpacking trauma (if you want a visual, Pediaa shares a cohesive breakdown of the differences on their website).* Due to experiencing racism and its many forms, many of us have been affected more than we realize. We all show this impact in many ways. Some of us feel constant anxiety during even the most basic daily functions of life, some of us have begun to isolate and avoid the things we used to enjoy, and some of us are constantly feeling charged up and angry for what seems like no reason at all. All these versions of impact can be symptoms of PTSD and CPTSD, and we all deserve to be able to acknowledge these pieces of ourselves without shame and, over time, learn skill sets to help us to reduce the symptoms of racialized trauma. Collective liberation requires acknowledgment without shame and forward movement with intentional and healing practices for individuals and communities.

Post-traumatic stress disorder is often diagnosed in individuals who have been through a severe experience such as an accident, a war, sexual assault, or even a naturally occurring disaster such as an earthquake or hurricane. Symptoms of PTSD might include irritability, emotional detachment, severe anxiety, insomnia, flashbacks, isolation, and more, and treatment can include things like cognitive behavioral therapy (CBT), medication management, Eye Movement Desensitization and Reprocessing (EMDR), and spiritual practices.†

When Reena became pregnant, Hilary began to have flashbacks about her own childbirth experience when she delivered Reena. During that experience, Hilary was ignored and disrespected, and she almost lost her life as a result of the racism and discrimination she was experiencing

---

* Hasa, "Difference Between PTSD and Complex PTSD," Pediaa, accessed June 15, 2022, https://pediaa.com/difference-between-ptsd-and-complex-ptsd/.

† "What Is Posttraumatic Stress Disorder (PTSD)?," American Psychiatric Association, accessed June 15, 2022, https://www.psychiatry.org/patients-families/ptsd/what-is-ptsd.

during a very critical and vulnerable moment in her life. When Reena announced her pregnancy, Hilary was more than excited about being a grandmother but also could not deny the symptoms of PTSD that she was experiencing, such as irritability, anxiety, and nightmares. Before Reena's pregnancy announcement, Hilary felt fine and thought she was completely healed from her negative experience. Unfortunately, Hilary did not receive therapeutic care when these symptoms began, though she knew it would be vital to her well-being after Reena's death.

CPTSD is much less talked about but is important to know and understand. Unlike PTSD, CPTSD is caused by prolonged or chronic stress. Long-term trauma can look like ongoing childhood abuse or neglect, living in a war zone, or being abused by a caretaker or an intimate partner. People experiencing CPTSD have some symptoms of PTSD but also additional symptoms that could include problems with their self-esteem, lack of emotional regulation, detachment/dissociation, mistrust, difficulty in relationships, and physical symptoms such as dizziness and nausea that aren't related to any medical issues. Treatments for CPTSD can include the same treatments as PTSD but usually last for a longer time.*

During the birth of his child, Jarrod constantly battled with speaking up for himself and Reena as decisions were made that he didn't always agree with. He struggled with being seen but not heard due to his fear of being seen as an aggressor and possibly being removed from Reena's side. This fear had come from constantly, directly or indirectly, experiencing police violence and abuse in his life. As mentioned above, living in a war zone can cause long-term trauma and lead to a diagnosis of CPTSD. A war zone is defined as an area marked by extreme violence. This is exactly what Jarrod experienced most of his life growing up poor and in an area that was highly surveilled by non-BIPOC police who believed it was an "us versus the community"

---

* Evangelina Giorou et al., "Complex Posttraumatic Stress Disorder," *World Journal of Psychology* 8, no. 1 (March 2018): 12–19, doi: 10.5498/wjp.v8.i1.12.

situation. That mindset resulted in the abuse of power from police officers, as well as multiple unwarranted shootings, arrests, and deaths. This upbringing resulted in CPTSD for Jarrod and later affected the way he was able to conduct himself during the birth of his child and death of his partner.

Somatic Pause: Uncovering Our Own Trauma

Many of you may recognize symptoms in yourself that have been reflected in Reena, Hilary, and Jarrod's experience, and that is OK. It is OK to acknowledge the pieces of you that may feel broken or uneasy.

In this next exercise, I would like you to pause for a moment and think of a traumatic experience you had over the last couple of years. This could be anything that popped into your mind when thinking about trauma as something that is too much, too soon, and too fast. As you are moving through this memory, take some deep breaths in through your nose and out through your mouth, pausing between each breath to recollect yourself and take notice of the sensations happening in your body.

Second, take some time to connect those sensations with emotions you are feeling and name those emotions without placing judgment on yourself for feeling the ways you feel. Do you feel anxious, angry, energized, stuck, or maybe even unusually calm or numb? What was your reaction to this experience when it happened? Did you cry, walk away, scream, lash out, say nothing, or go into people-pleasing mode, hoping to make everything better quickly? Try not to judge your response to the traumatic experience. Understand that your response is actually quite normal. Take several deep breaths and bring yourself into the present moment by looking around your space and naming items and colors that you see around your space. I also welcome you to pause for movement, journaling, or any other method of release and self-soothing if that is helpful.

Generational Trauma

I have been blessed to have been able to share time with my mother (La'Shayla), my grandmother (Mariam), my great-grandmother (Ardel), and my great-great-grandmother (Gladys) all together when I was younger. Currently, at thirty-three years old, I am still able to spend time with everyone but my great-great-grandmother Gladys who died in 2008 at the age of ninety-three. One thing for sure is all of us are spicy and sassy as all hell. But I have also realized in several ways how we have experienced similar traumas—all at different times in history but all very similar. I always wondered why that was or how could that even be, and during my ongoing study of trauma, I decided to read *It Didn't Start with You* by Mark Wolynn. I read in chapter 2, "The Generations of Shared Family History—The Family Body":

> The history you share with your family begins before you are even conceived. In your earliest biological form, as an unfertilized egg, you already share a cellular environment with your mother and grandmother. When your grandmother was five months pregnant with your mother, the precursor cell of the egg you developed from was already present in your mother's ovaries.
>
> This means that before your mother was even born, your mother, your grandmother, and the earliest traces of you were all in the same body—three generations sharing the same biological environment. This isn't a new idea: embryology textbooks have told us as much for more than a century. Your inception can be similarly traced in your paternal line. The precursor cells of the sperm you developed from were present in your father when he was a fetus in his mother's womb.*

---

* Mark Wolynn, *It Didn't Start with You: How Inherited Family Trauma Shapes Who We Are and How to End the Cycle* (New York: Viking, 2016), 25–26.

Reading this connected so many dots for me. Looking at my great-grandmother's generation (and this is obviously a generalization, as talking about an entire generation must be), the typical response to racism was to flee from it. My great-grandmother, who I call Nana, was born in 1937 and was raised on a farm owned by a white family where Nana and her family were sharecroppers in the deep south of North Carolina—Chadbourn, North Carolina, to be exact. I have asked my nana about her experience during that time because I could only imagine the racism and discrimination she was met with on a daily basis. To my surprise, when she talked about the non-BIPOC owner, she spoke about him being fairly nice and not giving her family a hard time. She even spoke about her community being a nice place to live, something I couldn't quite grasp because my brain could only feel the awareness of the "racism with no consequences" era she grew up in. She described life as being fairly easy as long as they stayed out of the way of the non-BIPOC people. Funny enough, she described her sister as being a bit of a rebel because she often crossed the lines of whiteness without much fear, something she herself wouldn't dare try. As Nana speaks of her childhood and the fond memories she has of her parents and her surroundings, I can literally feel the calm in my body that comes with living a simple life, but I can also feel the underlying fear of what could have happened to her if she rebelled and cross the racial lines at that time. There's something there that feels simple yet so complex underneath the surface.

By contrast, my grandmother, Mariam, was born in 1952, and her generation, as the first wave of civil rights leaders, wanted to knock shit down. My nana, her mother, has always described my grandmother as someone who didn't have a problem sharing her opinion and doing what she wanted to do regardless of the rules. Of course, that came with its downfalls, but it also came with a strength that is still evident in her until this day, something I tend to embody without realizing it. She grew up in a time when she had many, sometimes violent, incidents with non-BIPOC people, and it seemed to motivate her to push the limits along with fellow members of her generations. When I listen to her tell stories about her life, she mentions traveling and experiencing life in ways that my nana would have never dreamed or dared to live because she wanted to stay out of harm's way. She was surrounded by the voices of Martin Luther King Jr., Rosa Parks, Malcolm X, John Lewis, and organizations like the Black Panthers that made it clear Black people were no longer going to accept being treated unfairly and unlawfully. To this day, my grandmother will not settle for less than what she deserves and isn't afraid to put up a fight if it's necessary for vital change.

My mom was born in 1968, and in my opinion, my mom's generation seems to fall somewhere in between. There appeared to be a certain complacency with the advancements my grandmother's generation brought to the table. My grandmother's generation paved the way for more interracial experiences in life and in corporate and educational spaces. As racism became more covert, and as things like job opportunities improved, Black people became more accepting of the more silent and less loud forms of racism. For example, when my mother became an adult, she was able to get a stable job, which she recently retired from, and she was grateful. With that position came explicit and implicit bias, but at that time, racism was accepted as being a part of the normal, as long it didn't affect the money she was able to bring home to care for myself and our family. My nana and my grandmother were proud of her and still are, but I often wonder about how these unresolved experiences with racism affected the way she saw herself and the way she raised me.

On my path to becoming an adult, keeping a position was often a topic of discomfort between her and me. In my twenties, I would change companies and positions every year or so for a host of reasons, often including racism, understanding that these companies were not loyal to me, nor did they care about my well-being. I remember feeling this fight between my mom's messaging of "find a steady job that you can retire from" and my own messaging of "fuck that shit, I'm not staying anywhere I'm not wanted"—but always understanding that her messaging was from her experience and the ways she had to exist to survive at the time.

My mom's generation is not wrong—but it's not good enough either. I have been able to build my business as a Black queer nonbinary woman, and that is a blessing that was fought for, and I honor the work my ancestors did. But then again, there's intersectionality— I'm a dark-skinned Black woman with a fair amount of education, so I have a mix of privileged identifiers, but my friends and family who don't have the same privileges are still struggling in the mud. They can't get an education, a good job, a safe space, a day in which they are not violated. I can't turn my back on that even if it isn't my experience. Their trauma is my trauma.

Moving Through Trauma

As my generation, and most people reading this book, have experienced, we are all carrying many personal experiences that include racialized trauma as well as traumas around our bodies, our childhood, our daily existence, and more. We are carrying not only the weight of our personal trauma but also the weight of our ancestors, some who have made us proud with their ongoing strength through existences that required unbelievable resilience and some who have not made us proud because of their actions that have created the racial divide we now exist in.

It's important to emphasize that when specifically speaking about racialized trauma, it exists in all of us. BIPOC people have experienced present-day and generational racialized trauma through consistently having to fight to be ourselves. Our ancestors were conquered and forced to comply with colonization in order to survive, and this has led to losing parts of our culture, being constantly devalued, and seeing the effects of stress on our mental and physical health. The mental and physical effects of ongoing racialized trauma in BIPOC folks can look like the BIPOC individual who has cut themselves off from the world, but it can also look like the BIPOC activist who is constantly on the front lines while their health and well-being take a steady decline because rest never feels accessible or available when your community is suffering and, unfortunately, dying. For non-BIPOC people, racialized trauma shows up in the ways many non-BIPOC are aiming to hold on to white supremacy through permanently being in fight mode when whiteness is no longer centered and equality and equity are being pushed as the new way of existing. As BIPOC people are gaining more opportunities to influence change, many non-BIPOC people are aiming to conquer and destroy BIPOC communities through various actions such as threatening physical harm and aiming to hold systemic levels of control. Some non-BIPOC people are also paralyzed and sitting in silence, which can be just as harmful as the violent non-BIPOC individuals, but these are all symptoms and outcomes of racialized trauma living in all our bodies.

When I look at my own lineage, I can see the through line between my experiences and those of my mother, my grandmother, and my nana. Even though we have all had different responses, we've all dealt with racism and its many faces. My nana chose to flee from it and find safety and solace in the resources that were available to her. My grandmother chose to deal with it head-on and cross the racial lines enough to create more expansiveness for Black people in the future. My mother chose to inhabit the new spaces that weren't available to the generations before her while dealing with racism in a way that kept her in fight mode, because the threat of racism was always there but it was best to create the appearance of conforming for her livelihood. I choose to confront racism, speak on it, and create structures where I am not reliant on racist systems for my livelihood and don't need to conform for acceptance. The ultimate truth is I am where I am today, and BIPOC communities are where they are collectively, because of the experiences (good and bad) and work of the generations before us. But now, how do we honor those experiences and utilize what has been learned to move through trauma instead of holding on to it?

The first step to moving through trauma is to understand that this process is not linear; it is ongoing and a journey of ups and downs. In order to move through trauma, we have to acknowledge the parts of ourselves that feel dark, heavy, and full of grief, as well as acknowledging the parts of ourselves that feel light, expansive, and healed. Both parts are necessary in honoring our pain, our growth, our happiness, and our overall humanity. To acknowledge these pieces of ourselves means that we also have to move intentionally and at a slower pace than the world requires us to move for survival. There's a reason why systems such as capitalism require us to move so fast from one place to another without thought, only focusing on our material abundance and financial success. The fast-paced movement creates an atmosphere where we aren't processing our realities or the feelings that may come up because of these realities. We aren't able to sit with and acknowledge the ways we feel excited or burdened. Without this acknowledgment, we are unable to move through trauma because we have no source to pull from and no health methods to activate, and therefore no progress is made toward collective liberation. I am asking you to slow down and *feel* as an act of resistance and a huge step toward the future we are creating for ourselves and generations to come.

Next, we must see this process as a practice that leaves room for the progress and setbacks we all will inevitably experience. This process of healing isn't one size fits all, which even extends to your own feelings: what works for you one day may not work for you the next. As I have been in the process of healing trauma, I have focused much of my effort on my attachment style. I have an avoidant-dismissive attachment style, meaning I tend to avoid emotional attachment to others due to past trauma in my life and learning to survive by being hyperindependent. In many ways, I have witnessed how this attachment style has helped me to survive, seemingly unscathed, in many experiences, such as toxic romantic relationships and racialized experiences I've had in corporate America. However, I also have witnessed how this attachment style has made me avoidant of love I deserved to receive and has even caused harm to others due to the way I can emotionally detach myself from anyone when I perceive a threat to be present. In the last few years, I have made conscious decisions to work through my trauma and move to a more secure attachment style, a more comfortable and trusting way of existing that leans into intimacy unless a *true* threat is present. However, in this process of healing, I have at points felt like I healed a behavior or thought process of mine just to see it pop back up again. I have also had times when I thought I figured out the formula to my healing process (therapy + reiki + prayer = healing, I thought), just to realize that formula no longer was true for me. What I realized is I need to see my healing as a practice, one that will include and exclude different healing modalities and ways of caring for myself. Also, instead of seeing setbacks as failures, I need to view them as times to pick up the pieces again and heal in a way that feels true for me going forward.

This next line could feel remote to you when you read it and may even cause some resistance in your body and in your thoughts. Another key factor to moving through trauma is inviting rest and play into your life. Pause and take notice of what your heart, mind, and body feel when thinking about inviting in these two components. Do you feel like you do or don't have the permission to rest and play? Does rest seem impossible? Does play seem childish or even minuscule? For me, rest and play feel like the complete opposite of who I am. I'm a pretty serious, focused, and action-oriented individual with many things on my plate to help move our community forward, but when I took a bird's-eye view, I realized being this person wasn't working for me. It was causing emotional instability, collapse, resentment, and an inability to slow down and acknowledge my own feelings, the first step to moving through trauma. I began to invite rest and play into my life as a necessary part of my ongoing healing process and my overall well-being. Rest can absolutely look like lying down and taking an hour-long nap, but that is not always accessible to everyone.

Rest can also look like canceling social events you aren't in the mood for, leaving your worries on your ancestor altar, or decreasing your sensory input by turning lights off, putting your phone down, and allowing yourself to escape in silence or music you love. Wondering how to include play in your life? The best example is to seek the expertise of children and their ability to find play even in the times of crisis. We take care of them, and they take care of us by embodying play on a level we tend to forget when we become adults and the world is coming at us fast. Play can include allowing yourself to be immersed in the imaginative worlds of the children around you, and it can also look like taking time to move your body for your own pleasure, spending time with people who live to hear you laugh, or reading a fantasy book that allows you to frolic in your imagination.

Moving through trauma will take effort, focus, and intention. Some days it will feel like the heaviest weight on your chest, making it impossible to fill your lungs with air, and other times it will come with a pureness and ease that feels automatic, just as easy as the way your heartbeat continues without thought. Healing won't be linear, and some days you will have to utilize twenty of the tools you have created for yourself before you can find one that gives you some sense of relief. The point is, that is OK. Notice how some of these somatic exercises throughout this book may resonate with you one day and feel like a bunch of baloney another day. That is OK, too. What matters most is your commitment to yourself, your healing, and, ultimately, the collective healing we are all working toward together. I want to personally thank you for your effort because your effort influences and enriches the healing of myself, my ancestors, and the world as a whole.

Somatic Exercise: Moving Through Trauma

In this chapter, we have discussed trauma, trauma responses, forms of racism, racialized trauma, generational trauma, and ways to move through trauma. Through the somatic exercises, you have begun to identify what trauma looks like to you, as well as to recognize trauma in your own lived experience, which we understand can show up in a multitude of ways based on your identities, culture, and more. In the last exercises of this chapter, I would like for you to identify active ways to create an ongoing healing practice that will include slowing down enough to acknowledge and feel your feelings (emotionally and physically), invite the ups and downs of this process, and include elements of rest and play.

For BIPOC Readers

As I stated before, many of the systems of oppression affect us by keeping us moving at a fast pace so we are unable to acknowledge or feel. In a larger context, this absence of feeling and being able to hear our thoughts keeps us away from being in touch with our power. Also, as positions of power become more visually Brown and Black, and as white accomplices support more equality and equity practices, it is easy to be distracted by non-BIPOC people using harmful speech and actions as a way of acting out as a response to seeing their power erode. In this next exercise, I would like you to actively reclaim your time, your energy, and your healing through the following steps. Understand that there is no battle to win if we aren't caring for the long-term sustainability of ourselves and our communities.

1. Look at your calendar for the week ahead.

2. Cancel anything that does not serve a positive purpose in your life (e.g., hanging out with a friend who will dump all their struggles on you without your consent).

3. Find one (or two) spaces in your calendar where you can insert rest and/or play into your schedule, even if it's only for a few minutes. Be intentional with this time and write out exactly what you plan to do. If it's a nap time, then great, but you are also welcome to bring in any form of rest or play that resonates with you. Play in makeup, draw on your bedroom wall, allow yourself to really let go!

4. Hold yourself accountable for following through with this time, and after you spend time resting or playing, answer the following questions.
   a. How did it feel to rest or play?
   b. What did your body feel like before and after?
   c. How can you continue this element of your ongoing healing practice?
   d. Feel free to write down anything else that may come up for you.

For Non-BIPOC Readers

I would like you to take part in the exercise of rest and play above, yet in a conscious and balanced way, making sure not to use rest and play as an excuse for inaction. However, understand that your context and need for this exercise is different from that of BIPOC people. It is important for non-BIPOC people to realize that they are participating in racist systems and have a privileged place in these systems. Building awareness of your own power and privilege and how you are perpetuating those systems is key to moving through trauma. This is where white guilt can enter and dampen the pace of moving through the racialized trauma experienced and into action due to the frozen feeling of guilt.

None of us are the creators of this system—we are generations later. None of us have started this, but all of us can work to dismantle it. In fact, it is the job of non-BIPOC people to ensure they are working on deconstructing these systems at all times. If not, through your passivity and inaction, you're still a part of it and still perpetuating it. Acknowledging it and sitting in your guilt is not enough—it doesn't actually solve anything. Processing racialized trauma is collective, and that also means you must include rest and play as well, in order to promote your long-term wellness and sustainability, while taking daily action to create more equitable spaces for BIPOC communities. Let go of the guilt, create an ongoing plan of action, and consistently be on the path to healing and liberation.

6

HEALTHY COMMUNITY, HEALTHY PARENT, AND HEALTHY BABY

The greatness of a community is most accurately measured by the compassionate actions of its members.

—Coretta Scott King,
speech delivered in 2000 at Atlanta service
summit in honor of her late husband

TYPICALLY WHEN WE talk about unhealthy communities, we begin by bringing attention to the people in the communities, such as drug addicts, impoverished people, single parents, and other groups, who we may deem as unhealthy or not assisting the community with progressing into a healthy environment for its members, especially children and young adults. From there, we may start to name other problematic conditions in these unhealthy communities, such as failing education systems that are heavily involved in the school-to-prison pipeline, medical systems that do not adequately provide for the community members, the presence of food deserts, the high rates of police presence and violence, lack of support for people experiencing mental health and/or substance issues, unsafe homes and neighborhoods, and so much more. Notice that many of these conditions in unhealthy communities are usually blamed on the people of these communities. For example, many think that if poor people would stop being lazy, then they could live a higher-quality life. Some people think those dealing with substance abuse are to blame for higher police presence and violence because they have chosen to use substances that are dangerous and mind altering. Even in our many failing educational systems, children are blamed for their disruptive behavior and seen as the problem that has to be removed. There's an overall mindset that healthy parents and babies create a healthy community. It is my belief that this path is incorrect, and instead healthy communities create healthy parents, who then create healthy babies.

People affected by racism, bias, discrimination, trauma, and other involuntary harm of any kind cannot be both the victim and the source of the problem. Using the examples above, poor people have been affected by the violent inequities of capitalism, a lack of resources, and a lack of support, all of which have pushed them into unhealthy communities where survival is the daily struggle. People dealing with substance abuse have been affected by a lack of education and resources, as well as a lack of access to reputable and high-quality substance recovery programs that sometimes take days, weeks, and even months to find an open bed in. In our failing education systems and intensified school-to-prison pipeline, children in unhealthy communities are dealing with high-stress environments and a lack of readily available trauma-informed resources as well as resources appropriate to assist with neurodivergence and other disabilities. Children are being criminalized at young ages, and schools are calling the police on elementary students instead of aiming to understand the origins of their behaviors and their needs that are going unmet. How could they not be angry and experience outbursts without the necessary support all children should have?

> *The struggle is real. Yet when girls strike back against this fatigue, society casts them as deviant—as disruptive to the order of a (supposedly race- and gender-neutral) social structure without consideration of what might be fueling their agitation.*
>
> —Monique Morris, *Pushout: The Criminalization of Black Girls in Schools**

Taking this idea back to the topic of birth and the Black perinatal and infant mortality crisis, many hypothesized that the causes of these outcomes were factors such as Black birthing people not getting to prenatal care early enough, not eating properly, not making enough money, and other assumptions that placed blame and responsibility on the Black birthing parent for the death of themselves and potentially their child as well. However, as we have repeated many times

---

* Monique W. Morris, *Pushout: The Criminalization of Black Girls in Schools* (New York: The New Press, 2015).

in this book, after many studies the conclusion has been that racism and discrimination within the community surrounding Black birthing people and infants were to blame for these outcomes, not the Black birthing people themselves. This means that in order for Black birthing people and infants to have better outcomes, the community around them would have to shift entirely. Healthy communities, healthy parent, healthy baby.

So what does a healthy community consist of? To answer this question, it is important to consider the reason reproductive justice was created. It was created because marginalized communities were not being supported in second-wave feminism and could not relate to the demands that were being made by mostly non-BIPOC women. During second-wave feminism, non-BIPOC cis women fought for abortion access while BIPOC communities were fighting for access to health care. Non-BIPOC cis women also fought for equal pay while BIPOC communities were fighting to have access to employment opportunities. Although second-wave feminism efforts were legitimate, they did not speak to the more critical needs of BIPOC communities. Marginalized communities needed more to create the healthy communities that should be available to all. A healthy community goes beyond health care and education and instead creates a well-rounded holistic approach to creating community by including important factors such as community service and safe physical environments for all. To create a healthy community that is reproductive-justice based and trauma-informed, the community must include quality health care, quality education, adequate employment and job-training opportunities, safe and healthy environments, public transportation, civic engagement, arts and culture, and nutrition and recreation.

Quality Health Care

Quality health care is accessible health care, such as medical care and mental health care, that is based in patient-led and patient-centered care, ongoing anti-racism training/practices, and trauma-informed care principles, as well as a transparent accountability system. This should also include providers who come from a variety of communities and who have experiences similar to those they serve. In our current medical system where racism and discrimination exist, there has been proof of racially concordant care and culturally competent care creating a more positive experience and outcome for birthing people who are part of marginalized communities. Although many medical systems are beginning to increase their anti-racism and trauma-informed care principles education, there has yet to be a universal accountability system that can hold providers and other medical professionals accountable for negative outcomes that could have been avoided. A transparent accountability system with consequences, restorative correction plans, and more would protect everyone, especially Black birthing people and their children. As we continue to experience Black birthing people becoming victims of the racism and discrimination in health care systems, we see more public outrage but have yet to see a universal system that will hold health care providers accountable for their actions and, many times, inactions. Perhaps we can't miraculously change implicit and explicit bias, but creating systems of accountability and actively requiring consequences can assist with making health care providers more intentional and aware of their actions, while also creating an understanding that Black bodies are valuable and deserving of quality medical care.

Quality Education

Quality education refers to accessible education on all levels of the education system, including resources for different styles of learning, education-focused options, and the resources needed to care for the emotional and mental needs of all students. Again, educators should also be of the community and have a transparent accountability system that includes transformative and restorative justice practices for teachers and other professionals, as well as for students. It is also important to provide quality education to community members across many avenues, such as financial literacy, nutrition, pregnancy, general health, comprehensive sex education, and more. Traditionally, education stops after leaving the school system, meaning community members have to lean on authority figures to give them unbiased education, which we all know is not always possible because of the power structures built within the educational system that prioritize non-BIPOC bodies and criminalize BIPOC children at their point of entry. Having accessible education across the lifespan of a community member empowers the community to learn on their own and have a collaborative approach to working with professionals, such as doctors, police officers, and therapists. This approach to education would lead to more well-rounded and culturally competent content that also acknowledges the expertise of lived experiences and learned knowledge.

Adequate Employment and Job-Training Opportunities

Adequate employment and job-training opportunities mean employment that includes good wages, benefits, work hours, and accommodations for all community members seeking employment. Suitable employment also includes paid job-training opportunities, reasonable commuting distance, and opportunities for advancement. For birthing people, this topic cannot be avoided, especially with its connection to reproductive justice. Again, reproductive justice supports a birthing person's ability to have or not have a child, and income has always been highly connected to this decision for many. In 2012 *The Nation* reported "a quarter of all 'poverty spells'—falling into poverty for two months or more at a time—begin with the birth of a child."* Unfortunately, health care, housing, and other basic human rights have become linked to employment, meaning if a person does not have a job at a company that can provide living wages and benefits, they may be unable to access their basic human rights to having basic needs met. We know this to be unjust, but until there is a major shift in that connection, suitable employment and job-training opportunities are essential to the wellness of the community—the parents and the children of the community who need good wages, benefits, and more to maintain their mental, physical, and financial health for themselves and their families.

Safe and Healthy Physical Environments

Physical environments, such as homes, schools, business, and nature sites, should be safe, healthy, and clean. All physical spaces should have safe running water, electricity, accessible restrooms, and other resources that are necessary for community members. For birthing people this is essential, as many navigate wanting to feel safe and secure during a very physically vulnerable time in their lives and also a time when they are constantly visiting places such as the doctor's office to get themselves and their family ready for the next phase of their lives. When I attended my first reproductive justice conference, I decided to go to a session about reproductive justice and water. The

---

* Bryce Covert, "Too Often, a New Baby Brings Big Debt," *The Nation*, May 15, 2012, https://www.thenation.com/article/archive/too-often-new-baby-brings-big-debt/.

facilitator, an Indigenous birth worker, opened the space by having us pass around a bowl of water and extend gratitude to water and the ways it supports our lives. That is where I learned about many Indigenous birthing people not having access to safe water to drink and its impact, including difficult pregnancies, poor birth outcomes, and even infant death.

Public Transportation

Every community should have accessible, safe, and affordable public transportation that is available to all 24/7 and includes different types of options, such as buses, trains, and light rails, with accommodations for disabled community members. When I lived in San Diego, there were birthing centers that took Medicaid but still did not have the amount of Medicaid patients they were hoping to reach. On the other hand, I also knew many birthing people on Medicaid who wanted an out-of-hospital birth experience (births taking place at a birth center or in the birthing person's home) but were not able to sign up with the available birthing centers because of the distance and lack of affordable or timely transportation, or because many health insurers do not cover out-of-hospital births. A few shifts in the public transportation system of San Diego would have allowed more birthing people, especially those who are marginalized, to experience a different birth experience that research has shown to have a positive outcome for Black birthing people and their infants.

Nutrition

Food deserts are regions where people have limited access to healthy and affordable food. According to the USDA's Food Security Report, in 2019 an estimate of 10.5 percent of the US population was food insecure.* Community members must have accessible, healthy, and affordable food options (grocery stores, farmers markets, restaurants, food delivery services, etc.) that focus on making local food resources accessible and available to community members. They need well-rounded food and health education that meets people where they are with practical information and easy-to-understand language instead of promoting typical diet types. Accessible nutrition creates healthier bodies for all people of all age ranges, but especially birthing people. Receiving the essential nutrients that come from quality and accessible food creates birthing bodies that are healthier, stronger, and better able to deal with potential illness, and this ability can be transferred into their children.

Arts and Culture

Communities should have consistent community-led celebrations of the local arts and cultures of their members through activities such as music, dance, spirituality, theater, painting, and architecture. A connection to local arts and culture can improve stress levels, increase joy, connect community members, connect youth to their culture, and so much more for all people, including birthing people.

Civic Engagement

Civic engagement involves community-member advocacy focused on influencing change for the community led by those who are most impacted. Consistent civic engagement is open to all community members—from diverse races, economic statues, and political views—and in accessible ways, such as allowing in-person and virtual options.

---

* Alisha Coleman-Jensen et al., "Household Food Security in the United States in 2020," US Department of Agriculture, Economic Research Report Number 298, 3, https://www.ers.usda.gov/webdocs/publications/102076/err-298.pdf?v=7786.

For birthing people, civic engagement can be very vital in conversations about hospital policy, new resources for birthing people, and lactation policies, as well as heavy topics such as understanding why a birthing person has died during labor and what actions are going to be taken as a result of the death. People of the community deserve to be at the table for all the things that may positively or negatively impact the community.

Community Service

Community service initiatives should be led by the community members that help connect the community, bring social awareness to the initiatives in the community, and maintain the health of the community. Community service can look like an accountant providing tax services for a local nonprofit. It can also look like a community member assisting a new birthing parent with their household as they navigate creating systems around their child and new phase of life. The beauty of community service is it can benefit both people taking part in the service—the person giving and the person receiving—and it also creates opportunities for community members to fill in the gaps of care that need to be filled immediately and consistently.

Recreation

Quality recreation means easy access to affordable, fun, and health-increasing activities such as outdoor, physical, social, musical, and more. All types of recreational activities should also be accessible to community members of all physical and mental abilities. Recreational activities decrease stress, increase life satisfaction, create learning opportunities, increase self-esteem, and more. Of course, recreational activities are essential for the well-being of birthing people but are not always accessible or affordable.

*

These pillars working together create the healthy communities that we all deserve. More important, these factors take the blame off the community members who may be presently existing in unhealthy communities and build the framework and resources needed to start working toward a healthier community. They also provide members with resources to address their health and well-being holistically and from an empowered approach instead of with the common feeling of being told that they are not the expert on themselves and their experiences. This shift to building healthy communities isn't an easy one, but it is not impossible. It is a new approach for the new world we are creating through collective action and liberation.

Trauma-Informed Care Principles

Throughout this book, we have talked about the importance of trauma-informed care as a healing modality that is a necessary requirement in any community. We have also talked about the benefits of trauma-informed care such as creating a pathway for community members to be collaborative in their health care while developing trusting relationships with health care providers and promoting mental and physical well-being to all community members through accessible and culturally humble resources. Trauma-informed care can also go beyond health care interactions and into our personal lives by creating safer containers to acknowledge positive and negative experiences while intentionally creating support systems and tools.

Exercise: Health and You

Go back to a time when you interacted with a health care provider. This could be during any kind of a planned or unplanned medical visit or even perhaps a time you were present to assist with the medical visit of someone else, such as a child or a parent. Perhaps go with the first interaction that comes to mind. Why do you think this experience stood out to you, and how did you feel about that experience? What physical sensations do you feel in your body when recalling this medical visit, and what do these sensations tell you about your experience? Are any of these sensations aligned with sensations you feel when recognizing trauma, or do these physical sensations align with sensations that present themselves when you feel cared for? Did you leave feeling heard and cared for? Did you feel ignored, not valued, or any other negative feelings? Did you have mixed feelings? If it is helpful, write out your thoughts and feelings about this experience and any detail that sticks out to you during this exercise.

A major part of being able to give trauma-informed care is understanding the six trauma-informed care principles. These principles were created to serve as a framework for how service providers and systems of care can work to reduce the likelihood of retraumatization. Originally there were five principles: Safety; Trustworthiness and Transparency; Peer Support; Collaboration and Mutuality; and Empowerment, Voice, and Choice. In recent years an additional and necessary principle has been added: Cultural, Historical, and Gender Issues.*

SAMHSA (Substance Abuse and Mental Health Services Administration) explains the principles of trauma-informed care,† which I have clarified through the additions of my examples.

---

* Infographics, "Infographic: 6 Guiding Principles to a Trauma-Informed Approach," CDC, accessed June 15, 2022, https://www.cdc.gov/cpr/infographics/6_principles_trauma_info .htm.

† SAMHSA's Trauma and Justice Strategic Initiative, "SAMHSA's Concept of Trauma and Guidance for a Trauma-Informed Approach," Substance Abuse and Mental Health Services Administration, June 2014, https://store.samhsa.gov/sites/default/files/d7/priv /sma14-4884.pdf.

Safety

- "Throughout the organization, staff and the people they serve . . . feel physically and psychologically safe."
- Example: During Reena's experience, no one seemed to feel safe in the hospital space. Signs of an individual feeling safe can include feeling physically secure, feeling in control of their experience, and having the ability to speak their truth (including criticism) without fear of judgment or punishment. If Reena, Hilary, and Jarrod felt safe, there could have been more dialogue, more control over their birthing process choices, and an ability to voice their concerns and criticism knowing their words would be heard and valued.

Trustworthiness and Transparency

- "Organizational operations and decisions are conducted with transparency with the goal of building and maintaining trust with clients and family members, among staff, and others involved in the organization."
- During Reena's birth experience, she was told that a cesarean section was her next option because the hospital had a policy that stated any birth longer than thirty-six hours was an automatic cesarean section. Neither Dr. Smith nor Samantha took the time to explain the reasoning for this policy, and they also did not provide any unbiased scientific research that would assist Reena and her family in making an informed decision. If Reena and her family had received the explanation as well as the unbiased information, trust between Reena and her medical providers could have increased, and an informed patient-led decision could have been made.

Peer Support and Mutual Self-Help

- These "are key vehicles for establishing safety and hope, building trust, enhancing collaboration, and utilizing [peers'] stories and lived experience to promote recovery and healing."
- According to Mental Health America, "peer supporters offer emotional support, share knowledge, teach skills, provide practical assistance, and connect people with resources, opportunities, communities of support,

and other people."* In the birth world, one of the main peer support options is obtaining a doula. A doula could have provided Reena with education, resources, and ongoing emotional and other support during her birthing process. It is important to note that Reena could have obtained a doula on her own, but doulas are not always accessible for many reasons. It is important for the medical system to also provide Reena with ways to obtain a doula through different avenues, especially if accessibility is a barrier.

Collaboration and Mutuality
• "Importance is placed on . . . demonstrating that healing happens in relationships and in the meaningful sharing of power and decision-making. The organization recognizes that everyone has a role to play in a trauma-informed approach. . . . 'One does not have to be a therapist to be therapeutic.'"
• During Reena's birthing process, Dr. Smith did not have a great bedside manner. He was distant and seemed to talk at Reena and her family, instead of talking with them. Reena's experience could have been improved if Dr. Smith had made an attempt to talk to Reena and her family and thoroughly explain his concerns during her labor, as well as explain the hospital policies affecting Reena's outcome. With a collaborative approach, Reena, Hilary, and Jarrod would have felt empowered to make decisions based on the information explained by Dr. Smith and their opinion of how they would have liked to move forward with that information. A collaborative approach would have also shifted power to its rightful owner, Reena, instead of Dr. Smith and others seemingly maintaining more power than Reena over her own body and experience.

Empowerment, Voice, and Choice
• "Throughout the organization and among the clients served, individuals' strengths and experiences are recognized and built upon. The organization fosters a belief in the primacy of the people served, in resilience,

---

* "What Is a Peer?," MHA: Mental Health America, accessed June 15, 2022. https://www.mhanational.org/what-peer.

and in the ability of individuals, organizations, and communities to heal and promote recovery from trauma. . . . Clients are supported in shared decision-making, choice, and goal setting."

• During the birth of Reena's child, a hospital policy was brought to her and her family's attention. This hospital stated that any birthing person experiencing labor longer than thirty-six hours was subject to a cesarean section. During the cesarean section, her baby survived but she passed away. Although labor is a very common and normal experience, every labor experience is one of a kind. When policies are created to standardize a birthing person's unique labor process, that birthing person loses their ability to choose their own path. There's no way to tell what outcome Reena would have had if things were different, but had her choices been based on her unique labor process, instead of following a one-size-fits-all hospital policy, different decisions might have been made.

Cultural, Historical, and Gender Issues

• "The organization actively moves past cultural stereotypes and biases; . . . leverages the healing value of traditional cultural connections; incorporates policies, protocols, and processes that are responsive to the racial, ethnic, and cultural needs of individuals served; and recognizes and addresses historical trauma."

• During Reena's birth experience, Hilary was experiencing trauma symptoms based on her own traumatic birth years ago and her belief that Black women are not prioritized in the health care system, especially during birth. Jarrod was also experiencing trauma related to being a Black man in the United States and carrying the weight of not wanting to be seen as a danger to the care team, while also feeling inadequate because he wasn't able to code-switch the way Hilary and Reena were. Hilary and Jarrod were both affected by race-based trauma connected to their personal experiences, as well as the common experiences of people in their culture. Trauma-informed care principles would have created a space for these traumas to be acknowledged by the hospital and the professionals, such as Dr. Smith and Samantha, therefore creating a safer space for all involved.

Exercise: Health and You (continued)

When reviewing the six trauma-informed care principles, do you wish certain principles would have been applied more to your experience? How would that have shifted your experience and outcome? Do you feel these principles were active in the interaction, and how did the principles assist in creating a positive experience for you?

For myself when I think about a medical visit, I first think of any interaction I had with a specific non-BIPOC cardiologist. I went to him after being hospitalized and out of work for several weeks due to an unstable heart rate that increased to the point of feeling faint when I stood up and often not being able to lower my heart rate for, at one point, several days. To put it quickly, after I explained my health complications to him, he told me I was probably dehydrated, advised me to drink more water, and dismissed everything I had to say after his advice. I still feel hot in my chest when I think about that time. Two years later, I met with an Indian cardiologist due to still having ongoing episodes of an unstable heart rate. He listened to me and assessed me while explaining everything he was doing, and I left the office with a diagnosis of inappropriate sinus tachycardia (IST) and a treatment plan with options. As I write about it, I can feel the weight lifting off my chest and a warmth building in my body. The second cardiologist I saw applied many of the trauma-informed principles, such as mutuality and collaboration and trustworthiness and transparency, simply by listening to me and understanding I am the expert of my body.

If you are a provider of any kind, what principles do you need to apply to your work more? Where can you improve in your care, and what impact will that have on the individuals you serve? We all have space to improve, and there is no shame in that.

Investing Versus Reinventing

I would be remiss if I didn't mention the many organizations, especially BIPOC organizations, that have been doing this work of creating accessible and trauma-informed resources in the journey of establishing healthy communities. For some of you, your job will be to create new resources that do not currently exist in your community. However, many of you will instead need to invest your money, time, or energy into current resources making change and doing the work instead of reinventing the wheel. Remember, we make more change collectively than we do individually, and that truth applies deeply to the goal of creating healthy communities, healthy parents, and healthy babies.

Kimberly Seals Aller, the writer of *The Big Letdown: How Medicine, Big Business, and Feminism Undermine Breastfeeding*, created the Irth (Birth Without Bias) app. Irth is an app that allows individuals to rate their interactions with perinatal and pediatric providers, creating a space for community reviews done by and for the Black and Brown community of birthing people. Reviews can be left from the prenatal period to the child's first year after birth, and reviews can be searched by filters such as race, income, gender, and sexual orientation. Also, the questions being asked of reviewers go further than name, location, and ratings from 1 to 10. Irth asks questions about feeling respected by the doctor, reasons for holding back from asking questions or discussing concerns, and whether something about the birthing person, such as race, gender, marital status, or ethnicity, greatly impacted the care received. Birthing people, their partners, and birth workers are also able to leave reviews in the Irth app. The data collected is being used to create institutional change, and specific symbols show Irth users where the death of a birthing person or infant has taken place. Irth has created a database that is free and easily accessible for Black birthing people to find information and provide feedback in a way that has not been possible before.

Indigenous Women Rising (IWRising) was established in 2014 by Rachael Lorenzo (Mescalero Apache/Laguna Pueblo/Xicana) to raise awareness and advocacy for Indigenous women who were being denied access to Plan B by the Indian Health Services. Since its creation, IWRising has aimed to "create space for indigenous people to tell their own stories on their terms as an act of resistance, self-love, and love for [their] ancestors and family." IWRising cares about issues such as access to abortion, culturally congruent perinatal health care, comprehensive mental and behavioral health, and sex education. Current programming includes an abortion fund, a midwifery fund, and a sex education program.*

In Tkaronto (colonially known as Toronto), an IBPOC community-run and -operated collective by the name of Ocama Collective provides traditional and holistic birthing support for queer and IBPOC communities. The key goal for the Ocama Collective is to "facilitate a safe space for 2S [two spirit], trans, queer, non-binary, genderqueer, and agender folx, to fully engage in pregnancy and birth care that is self-directed, holistic, and satisfactory." (IBPOC purposely places the *I* first to emphasize Indigenous people, and *folx* indicates acceptance of queerness and is used to create space for all birthing people.) The organization offers cost-supported care to reduce infant mortality, improve birth outcomes and satisfaction, and support parents through their journey physically, mentally, spiritually, and emotionally.†

BIPOC individuals and organizations (the list does not stop with the three we've discussed) have been doing the work and deserve to

---

* Indigenous Women Rising, "About Indigenous Women Rising," accessed June 15, 2022, https://www.iwrising.org/about-iwr.
† Ocama Collective, "Mission," accessed June 15, 2022, https://www.ocamacollective.com/about.

be invested in as they continue working toward healthy communities. Some additional resources are Postpartum Healing Lodge, founded by Raeanne Madison; Commonsense Childbirth School of Midwifery, founded by Jennie Joseph, LM; Birth Sanctuary Gainesville, founded by Stephanie Mitchell; Ancient Song Doula Services, founded by Chanel Porschia-Albert; and Black Mamas ATX, governed by the Black Mama Community Collective founded by Michele Rountree. The list of individuals and organizations doing the work of reproductive justice and creating trauma-informed care spaces for all is expansive and longer than most people realize.

It is now your time to pause and research the resources currently available in your community. Who is taking care of birthing people, especially marginalized birthing people? Are these spaces inclusive to all gender expressions and sexualities? Are the resources trauma-informed and continuing to work toward building safer spaces than what are usually provided to community members? Investing in your community does not only include financial resources. Investing can include filling a volunteer position, spreading awareness, and providing services such as tax preparation, administrative assistance, graphic design, website building, education, and childcare services. Remember, when we reinvent the wheel, we are taking away resources from community organizations that already exist, and we are causing a divide in the collective energy we can be putting toward sustainable and impactful change.

Using Reproductive Justice to Assess Healthy Communities

A step that can't be forgotten as we move toward healthy communities is setting a standard by which to assess the resources we are creating and investing in. The four pillars of reproductive justice are the standard and can be used to make sure we are all moving toward the same goal in an equitable and respectful way. As a reminder, the four pillars of reproductive justice are analyzing power systems, addressing intersecting oppressions, centering the most marginalized, and joining together across issues and identities. I will use my non-profit, For the Village, as the resource we will be assessing together to determine its compatibility with building and maintaining a healthy community.

For the Village was created in 2018 when I realized there weren't any community-based doula programs in San Diego, California. I was committed to assisting all birthing people, especially Black birthing people being directly affected by the Black perinatal and infant mortality crisis. I also realized many BIPOC and other margin-alized communities were looking for a place to train as a doula but either could not afford the available trainings or were discouraged because they did not see reflections of themselves in the training they attended. As of the end of 2021, we have trained 67 doulas of all races and identities, and we have served 236 birthing people in San Diego County.

As For the Village has continued to expand, I have regularly assessed our direction and mission using the four pillars of repro-ductive justice. This assessment has been key to our growth because it has kept us aligned with the mission of creating healthy communities, healthy parents, and healthy babies.

Analyzing Power Systems

In our work at For the Village, we are constantly analyzing power systems such as hospitals, social services, child protective services, and others—and that work will always continue to happen in our daily routine. However, it is important to now begin to see ourselves as not only a community resource but a power system within the community as well. Being a resource for the community comes with power, which consistently needs to be checked and assessed to be sure we aren't operating like the power systems we have negatively interacted with. What should a community-centered and community-led power system look like? It should include community governance, decision-making, and leadership—all executed by community members who have a vested interest in their community. It should also include accessible ways for community members to be a part of the resource, as well as equitable policies and practices.

For the Village welcomes and makes changes and improvements based on the feedback we receive from our doulas, as well as from the members of the community we serve. We have also increased access to our doula training by offering our training to community members for free while also paying our doulas for their work with our clients. Lastly, we have created policies and practices based on what has already existed, instead of aiming to completely reinvent, and we have edited and improved these practices as we have learned more through experience and community feedback. We have also happily accepted that we are not all-knowing and have remained open to what we can continue to build with our community and other aligned power systems within the community. For those who are not aligned with our mission, we have created boundaries in how we work with these systems. For example, we have committed to not being in direct partnership with hospital systems so we can remain community-based. However, when we do work with these systems, we interact respectfully while being sure to center our client's wants, needs, and experience.

Questions to ask:
- What does a new power structure look like for our community?
- Is our power system led and inspired by the community we are serving?
- Are our services, policies, and practices equitable and accessible?

- What additional power systems are we working with, and are they aligned with our mission? If not, what are the boundaries we have in place when working with these power systems?

Addressing Intersecting Oppressions

From the beginning of For the Village, we have always discussed intersectionality in our doula training. We understand that a lack of intersectionality can cause trauma for the clients we serve, as well as leave us unaware of critical information about these individuals. Through our years, we have also been able to give better care to our community members through the lens of intersectionality. In 2019 we received our first funding opportunity, which expanded our reach to at least one hundred clients per year. When we officially opened our services to the community, we saw a great number of Haitian immigrants signing up for our services, which was amazing! Prior to that rush of the Haitian community, we had served others in the Black community and had a good amount of knowledge of what our Black clients wanted and needed in our service, and we felt confident that this knowledge would easily translate to our Haitian immigrant population. We were wrong. Our Haitian immigrants were dealing with many different identities than our Black clients, such as language barriers, immigration status, homelessness, low to zero income, coming from an impoverished country, severe trauma, and more. We quickly learned that our Haitian clients and their intersections meant their needs were different and required a different approach. Without the knowledge of intersectionality, we would not have been able to provide the care and create the resources needed for our Haitian clients, such as written resources in French and Creole, Haitian doulas who understood their language and culture, transportation gift cards, clothing for both baby and parents, housing resources, and more. This is the beauty of intersectionality, and being aware of intersectional identities is ongoing work that creates more safety for our community members.

Questions to ask:
- How is intersectionality infused into the culture of an organization?
- Is intersectionality evident in all training materials and resources within the organization?
- How does the lack of intersectionality impact both the internal and external community members in the organization?
- How can intersectionality be used as a method of problem solving?

Centering the Most Marginalized

The Black perinatal and infant mortality rate has always been the focus of For the Village. We have also always been open to other community members and marginalized groups, including low-income families in San Diego County that would also benefit from having a doula but may not be able to afford the services. In regard to the perinatal and infant mortality crisis, Black birthing people are the most marginalized and have historically been underserved, although this crisis has been evident for generations. To center Black birthing people, any Black-identifying person is qualified to receive our doula services. The reason for this is research has shown that Black birthing people of any income status, education level, and so on are still at increased risk of dying during childbirth or within the first year after childbirth. In our opinion, centering the most marginalized means creating opportunity that is equitable and easy to access by decreasing as many of the barriers as possible.

Questions to ask:
- With our current mission, who is most affected by the issue we are addressing?

- Are our services equitable and easy to access with the least amount of barriers possible?
- Do we have the research and further information needed to understand the barriers presented to the most marginalized community?
- Are the members of the most marginalized group being represented, as well as being provided an accessible way to lead the actions of the organization?

Joining Together Across Issues and Identities

For the Village has not expanded in the ways it has over the years by itself. It's taken a mix of people from different races, genders, cultures, languages, job titles, power systems, religions, and more to make this organization grow! We all have had to push past our perceptions of each other to move toward the same goal of improving the Black perinatal and infant health disparities in San Diego County by providing community members with accessible full spectrum and trauma-informed doula care services. Another example of joining together across issues and identities is the beautiful combination of our doulas. San Diego is a mostly non-BIPOC community, but one thing that was important for us was to create a doula group that gave the TRUE expression of the many cultures and languages, spoken in San Diego County. I'm proud to say our doulas speak many languages, such as Spanish, Haitian Creole, French, Russian, and Persian. Joining together across issues and identities has allowed us to create a true reflection of the community, expand our reach, and gain necessary funding and other opportunities for the people we serve.

Questions to ask:
- What identities are currently present internally and externally in the organization?
- How are these identities honored (e.g., using inclusive language, spoken languages, etc.)?

- How do we deal with opposing views from internal and external community members?
- Do community members feel safe in our organization? Why or why not?

This method of assessment can be used to assess resources in our communities before we or others take part in the resource. This method of assessment can also be used for continued self-assessment of organizations we have created or are a part of. Using this method, along with understanding what a healthy community actually consists of, applying trauma-informed care principles, and investing in what already exists instead of reinventing the wheel, can and will push forward the positive change we are seeking in our communities while also creating safer spaces for the hard conversations and incidents that will undoubtedly happen as we create a new and improved future. One of the most beautiful things I have learned about reproductive justice is that it not only helps us to envision a new future but also helps us to move forward *into* that future, step by step, with standards that help us create and build upon the resources we need for a healthy community with healthy parents and healthy babies.

7

BIRTHING LIBERATION

As a black woman, my politics and
political affiliation are bound up with
and flow from participation
in my people's struggle for
liberation, and with the fight of
oppressed people all over the world
against American imperialism.

—Angela Davis, *LA Times* interview
"UCLA Red Lays Ouster Proceedings to Racism"

Y OUR PERSONAL LIBERATION is the key to collective liberation.

What does that even mean? It means that in order for us to free ourselves and our communities, to open our hearts, to be equal, to be equitable, to have a safe space for all of us—it starts with *you*. The individual leads to the collective.

Hurt people hurt people. It's an endless cycle of harm, and the only way out of it is through ongoing healing. People who are actively working on their traumas create space for others to do the same, and slowly, person by person, we can break this cycle. We can move into a space of self-awareness and empathy, a space free of both white supremacy and the "woke wars," until individual liberation becomes collective liberation. Until we are all free.

Collective liberation centers the healing of ourselves in order to mirror and model what's needed in our communities. It recognizes the personal work necessary to become a better version of ourselves without making it feel overwhelming; it's not as though one person is to blame for all of society's problems. Collective liberation recognizes that we are all part of a bigger system that has kept us out of touch with our inner awareness and more aware of external hierarchical systems that teach us to center power and privilege over community.

Our current world of white supremacy, capitalism, and patriarchy teaches us that polarity is needed for survival. We lean heavily into the masculine (strength, reason, and survival) while disregarding the feminine (healing, nurturing, and patience), and as a result we have been led into thinking we must always be better than someone else in order to be valuable. We must have more than someone else. We must see differences between people and create hierarchical systems based on those differences, and the people at the top must stay at the top by continuing to push the people at the bottom further and further down. Our personal value is measured by how much power and privilege we have, instead of by our ability to see each other as humans.

In order to maintain that power and privilege, we not only create division and hierarchy but also struggle with constant thoughts about what to do next to get or stay ahead, leaving less time and space to be in our bodies. This is intentional. Less time and space in our bodies causes less awareness of what we are actually experiencing, and so we fall further into systems of polarity.

We have all absorbed this messaging, and it has affected the way we treat ourselves and others. It has created a cognitive dissonance between our minds, our bodies, and our truths in ways that have created deep wounds for everyone, even the non-BIPOC folks who have consciously and subconsciously believed their overconsumption of power has been a benefit to their lives. It is not a benefit; it's actually a trauma response to a fear of scarcity.

There is good news. Our current ideologies and systems of oppression were created, and anything that has been created can be dismantled. I am welcoming you to dismantle what is and what has been and create a new way of existence.

Envisioning Collective Liberation

Let's take a moment to imagine what collective liberation would feel like deep inside of our bodies. What would it feel like to be able to be in community with people who are different from you—who have different lives, different cultures, different ways of existing—but to always feel valued for who you are? What would it feel like to be in community with people who share various parts of you, whether it's your race, your gender, or your sexuality, and be seen and held closely by those people? What would the world look like if we gave marginalized communities what they need to gain true equity, spanning from health care to economics? What if we knew that everyone giving birth would be safe, whether in a hospital or at home? What if instead of the police we had services that addressed the concerns that lead to violence and worked to heal communities restoratively? What if we all had the ability to live openly and freely and completely as ourselves, without persecution? Picture yourself in that world and really take in how it would feel to live there.

It all seems pretty great, right? But now take a look at how it would feel to do what is necessary to get there. If you are a non-BIPOC person, consider that, as a collective, white people will have to give up some of their wealth in order for it to be shared more equitably. Consider that you will have to give up feeling judgmental of others in order not to be judged yourself. Consider that you will have to give up your privilege if you are going to achieve equality.

When you think about collective liberation in this way, what sensations come up for you? Do you feel frozen? Do you feel open? Does your heart feel light or heavy? Do you feel resistant to giving up some of your power? Do you feel angry that this is even a conversation?

It is natural to feel resistance or even anger as you answer these questions in your mind and feel the responses in your body. This is an essential and major part of the process of transformation in our personal journey. It is human to feel resistance to a way of existence that is different from what you are used to. Change is hard, beautiful, and challenging, even when we know the change is for good. Can you recognize that feeling, hold a space for it, take away your judgment of yourself for feeling it, and simply breathe through it until an open space of possibility begins to become present in your mind and body? This is where knowledge of our nervous system is essential. This is the skill that we all need to contain and practice endlessly, sometimes on an hourly basis, in order to move from what is to what can be.

We have to be able to hold both feelings at the same time: our desire for collective liberation, and our resistance to it. Both are real and true, and we will never fully achieve collective liberation, no matter how much we want it, until we acknowledge our resistance and move through it.

So let's stay with that resistance a little longer. Achieving collective liberation requires centering the needs of those who have the least. If we create a new system that provides the 20 percent of the population with the resources they need, the lives of the other 80 percent will also improve because collective liberation is good for everyone. *But* this requires non-BIPOC folks to share the power and privilege that has been given to them from birth in an intentional way.

Upon reading that last sentence you may, consciously or unconsciously, feel some resistance for what feels like such a big ask. You may automatically default to giving donations to a local organization or volunteering your time to a purpose that seemingly affects BIPOC folks the most. You may also default to thinking about how nicely you treat Black and Brown people—and may believe that's enough.

It's not. You have to do more than that.

What will collective liberation require from non-BIPOC identifying people? It will require you to give up the power and privilege that has been given to you. Yes, you didn't sign up for this privilege of whiteness, and most of the time you don't even notice it—but you still have it, and you still have to give it up. You are required to intentionally dissect how the privilege of whiteness has given you a better chance of a better quality of life from birth, and to examine how that privilege has affected the people in your community who have not been afforded that privilege at birth.

As we've discussed in prior chapters, BIPOC infants die in childbirth at a rate two to three times that of non-BIPOC infants, for no other reason than racism and discrimination. Put simply, people are born with the privilege to survive and live beyond their first year of life just because they are born in white skin. There's also the school-to-prison pipeline, which impacts BIPOC communities the most. Currently, statistics put out by the ACLU indicate that Black students are arrested at higher rates than white students, are expelled or suspended 300 percent more often, and are 300 percent more likely to come into contact with the juvenile detention system within one year of being expelled or suspended.* The Racial Wealth Divide Report shows median non-BIPOC families have forty-one times more wealth than the median Black family and have twenty-two times more wealth than the median Latinx family.†

Is that a hard pill to swallow as a non-BIPOC person? Imagine the heaviness of reading these statistics while inhabiting a body that has been politicized, unprotected, and perceived as less valuable consistently over generations.

We cannot make the decision to decrease our power and privilege without accepting that privilege exists. Accepting these facts and metabolizing this information in your system will allow you to push beyond the fear and resistance that comes with moving toward collective liberation. It will help you deconstruct your power and privilege and rebuild yourself for the better in a way that doesn't use power as the main factor in your self-value. Because, whether you realize it or not, you have also consciously or subconsciously accepted the idea that your value is intrinsically tied to the power you have over marginalized and less privileged communities.

During this process, non-BIPOC people may feel overwhelmed with the feeling of not wanting to relinquish power, despite knowing that doing so will only create a better future for themselves, their family, and other people in this world. There may absolutely be feelings of resistance and resentment, which is a natural part of the process: "Damn, I can't have this power anymore. Damn, I have to give it up. Damn, I have to share it." What hardships or challenges will come

---

* "School-to-Prison Pipeline," ACLU, accessed June 15, 2022, https://www.aclu.org/issues /juvenile-justice/school-prison-pipeline/school-prison-pipeline-infographic.

† "Facts: Racial Economic Inequality," Inequality.org, accessed June 15, 2022, https:// inequality.org/facts/racial-inequality/.

with this shift when a non-BIPOC person can no longer navigate the world with the amount of power and privilege they have been using to their benefit? This level of risk is something that non-BIPOC bodies do not have much experience in, at least when compared to the bodies of BIPOC folks who have lived consistently at the tail end of privilege. The less privilege a person has, the less they are able to rely on the future for stability and comfort. That's a scary thought, and it is natural and normal to feel resistance to it. Of course you don't want to give up power. Accept and acknowledge that, because if you don't, you'll never be able to actually give it up.

Exercise: How Does Equity Feel?

For Non-BIPOC Readers

In my experience of working with non-BIPOC people aiming to embody anti-racism, it is easy to understand the concept of anti-racism and its components of equity and inclusion. However, it is harder to deal with the physical sensations of equity, which for some include feeling embodied expressions of positive feelings but for others can include embodied expressions of resistance, anger, and even fear. These feelings can make you question your goal of anti-racism because your feelings and physical sensations seem opposite of your personal goals, but this is where you push through in order to create capacity. Expanding your capacity will allow you to expand your ability to deal with your many feelings while creating a higher tolerance and acceptance of what it means and feels like to share power with BIPOC communities.

1. Find four of the same coin and place them in front of you.
2. Take these coins and hold all of them in your hand. Feel the weight of these coins, rub them, move them around, and notice what may be happening in your body as you hold all four of these coins.

3. Next, place the coins in front of you in a straight line. Look at them.
4. Slide one of the coins to the far right of you. Check in with yourself. Did any feelings come up? Any physical differences? Any resistance?
5. Now slowly slide another coin to the far left of you. How's your heart feeling? How's your breathing? Notice any changes?
6. Slowly slide another coin in front of you as far as it can go.
7. You should now be left with one coin. Pick it up and hold it. Have your feelings shifted from the first time you picked up the four coins? How does it feel to see the other coins but not be able to hold them? How does it feel to deliberately put the coins as far away from you as possible?

Ask yourself the following questions: How have I benefited from this power and this privilege that was given to me from birth? How have I used that power and privilege? What does it feel like for me to shift that power intentionally to another group, a group that has not been given the same access? How will I actively do that work while expanding my capacity for difference?

How does it feel to give up power? What happens to you somatically? What sensations do you carry? Be honest with yourself, for this is a major skill needed for collective liberation. We must develop the capacity to hold many feelings, both good and bad, with the reward of making the right choice at the end. Our current system of polarity forces us to choose a single emotion, and when we push our varying emotions away and fall into the habit of allowing ourselves to experience only one at a time, we have allowed this system to take away our ability to choose. I want you to feel *all* your feelings, to understand them and then deliberately choose the feelings that will move you along in our shared goal of collective liberation.

Through the journey to collective liberation, many non-BIPOC folks will ask themselves, "Will I truly be able to take on this challenge that will last a lifetime?"

The answer is yes. You can do it by remembering and choosing to focus on how collective liberation benefits *you* as well. We have to move away from the idea that anti-racism is a sacrifice for non-BIPOC folks and instead consider how collective liberation is also beneficial to non-BIPOC folks. We have to move away from the safety and passivity of being a non-BIPOC ally and into the humility, discomfort, and consistency it takes to be a non-BIPOC accomplice. Allies agree with the idea of collective liberation, while non-BIPOC accomplices move into BIPOC-guided action with a full understanding of how the systems that are failing BIPOC people are also failing non-BIPOC people.

White supremacy hurts us all. According to the Local and Regional Government Alliance of Race & Equity, when Black and Brown voters are constrained or suppressed, so are low-income white voters. Strategies designed to assist BIPOC youth with completing high school also benefit non-BIPOC youth, sometimes to an even greater degree. We talk so often about how reducing incarceration and recidivism rates help BIPOC males since they are the most-affected group, but obviously they also benefit *everyone* in the criminal justice system, including non-BIPOC people. These are just some instances of strategies and programs that were created to assist the most marginalized but are also beneficial to the collective.

Collective liberation will also offer non-BIPOC people a sense of belonging. There won't be any more worrying about having to be better than someone else or in competition with the world. They will be able to let their guard down. Right now, the experience of whiteness is limited. It may not be limited in resources, but non-BIPOC people are consistently drowning in fear of being without, fear of not being the dominant culture. They suffer daily in equating their value to what they have and not who they are.

Collective Liberation is the experience of recognizing the gifts in each and every person so that we can live in an elevated state as humans. For me, as a non-BIPOC cis woman, realizing that I'm not doing the movement for Liberation any service if I diminish myself or my gifts has been a wake-up call. When you are born into oppressive systems, you have to work at rewiring the response that for BIPOC people to rise, you need to suppress yourself. Collective Liberation allows for an experience as non-BIPOC that is also a healthy expression, a release from needing everyone to think the way you do. It's basically the opposite of everything our White Supremacy, Patriarchal, Neo-colonialist society would tell you!

—Andrea Berg, spiritual leadership coach[*]

Led by BIPOC, Enacted by Non-BIPOC

The personal liberation of BIPOC people means that we can exist in who we are and what we are and how we are at all times, not needing permission to be proud of ourselves, not needing permission to ask for what we need. No longer feeling imposter syndrome (which is the voice of the oppressor) and instead knowing that we are right where we should be, even when we are in spaces that historically have not welcomed us. Understanding that when we ask for what we need, we aren't asking for excess but are asking for exactly what we deserve. The personal liberation of BIPOC folks means that we, as well as the rest of the world, understand that joy is our birthright, and that joy includes being centered, having equity, and being in control of the ways we exist in the world.

---

[*] Andrea Berg, email to author, November 30, 2020.

Working on both personal and collective liberation gave me the permission I needed to push past the plateau I felt I had reached on my journey. It gave me permission to say no without feeling like I had to be forgiven, because my no was right for me. The pressure to not rest, to always keep striving for better, for more, for perfection, is one of the many ways I have internalized racism. It allowed me to decolonize my inner world, and watch my outer world follow suit. I integrate the principle of collective liberation into every aspect of my life— the things I choose to put into the world, the way I interact with people in my personal life, the way I communicate, are all done through the lens of collective liberation.

—Aaliyah Dailey, full-spectrum doula*

As a BIPOC queer nonbinary woman, I have always struggled with what liberation is for me. Is it the way I have freed myself in a world that doesn't always want to hear my voice, witness the beauty of my skin, or notice the natural texture of my hair? Is it measured in the times of rebelling against the dominant culture while knowing I was putting myself in situations to possibly be harmed? Is my liberation defined by those rare moments when I feel that I can be myself, existing in my body fully and completely?

What I've come up with is that all of the above are parts of my liberation, but that I am not fully free because I am not the dominant culture.

But that is not something I can change. I cannot *make* non-BIPOC folks give up their privilege. And yet somehow the responsibility for achieving collective liberation has always fallen on BIPOC shoulders. We have to carry the weight of being oppressed while also being expected to do the work to create and fight for an equitable environment. Think about it. Black and Brown people have always been the

---

* Aaliyah Dailey, email to author, November 20, 2020.

ones on the front lines, from Harriet Tubman to John Lewis to Stacey Abrams to the unnamed BIPOC individuals who have continued to put their literal bodies on the line because they understand their mission is bigger than themselves.

Imagine having no choice but to fight a war that you did not start, over and over, from generation to generation. And then imagine that the people whose ancestors did start the war got to *choose* whether they would like to participate in what they themselves have perpetuated. The mere fact of my existence as a BIPOC person threw me into this war the moment I was born. BIPOC folks are born into it, and we fight our way through our lives, losing people we cherish to police brutality and to everyday processes such as having a baby. That is the reality of racism. Its many forms impact everything from the racial wealth gap to our ability to literally live.

BIPOC folks did not create the systems of oppression and racism that currently exist, but historically we have been the ones to question, resist, and dismantle them. We have taken on the risk of our safety, health, and wealth time and time again because non-BIPOC people were too comfortable or too scared to do so. In the past, collective liberation has been framed as something non-BIPOC people can help with, instead of something non-BIPOC people are responsible for, with the assistance and direction of BIPOC folks.

Our current model of anti-racism work has to shift in order for true change to take place. Non-BIPOC people do not have the insight or lived experience of what it is like to be on the other side of racism, and so they must be led by the voices, experience, and expertise of BIPOC folks. This means non-BIPOC people have to step out of freeze, sometimes masked as confusion, and into deliberate action led by BIPOC people. They don't get to say they don't know what to do, and they don't get to give up when they've made a mistake. It also means that we need non-BIPOC people to show up physically in droves at protests and other forms of resistance. They have to put their bodies on the line, just as BIPOC bodies are every day.

They have to join the movement of collective liberation with a plan that's intentional, meaningful, and guided by BIPOC folks. That begins with understanding that the system that we have right now has been built with certain people in mind—and, specifically, with the intention of making sure whiteness is the dominant and superior culture. With that truth, we can begin to rebuild a system that includes everyone, and specifically prioritizes the BIPOC people who have been neglected in the system for centuries and up until our current time.

> I don't want an ally. Because an ally means you came here to help me. How are you helping me solve the problem you caused? Why aren't I helping you solve the problem you caused? What am I not the ally, and you the actor? Why is Blackness the responsibility holder and whiteness gets to be the helper?

—Sonya Renee Taylor*

Collective liberation is an understanding that we all need each other to truly be free. It breaks the concept of overt independence, which does not exist, and allows us to intentionally depend on each other in ways that are healthy, healing, and filled with opportunities for growth. Remember, your liberation is my liberation. One cannot happen without the other. You are not free until I am free. Collective liberation frees us from polarization, oppression, scarcity, and all the other harmful messages our current oppressive systems have led us to accept for so long. We do not need to continue to live in hierarchical systems; we can move instead to nonhierarchical communities that center people and relationships over rules and power. We can

---

* Sonya Renee Taylor, *The Body Is Not an Apology: The Power of Radical Self-Love* (Oakland, CA: Berrett-Koehler Publishers, 2021).

build this together with hard work, consistency, grace, and the goal of creating a safer world for generations to come.

We worry so much about the roles we play in generational trauma. What would it feel like to instead be a part of the mission of generational healing and, as Chanel Porschia-Albert says, of "instilling intergenerational hope"?*

Black Grief

As I have moved through and continue to move through my own journey of healing from racialized trauma and many other forms of trauma, I have begun to intentionally connect with the heavier part of myself that needs to be seen and needs energy and time dedicated to it. Prior to COVID-19 taking over in 2020, I was aware of grief because as a doula I have held the feelings of literal life and death for my clients. I'm familiar with grief through my own experiences as well, but for a lack of better words, COVID-19 and my personal lived experiences during the pandemic really knocked me on my ass. I had to deal with and embody in a way I never had experienced before, because the traumas came so fast, so soon, and way too frequently!

A couple years later, I am still working through the fog of experiencing back-to-back traumas. In the first leg of COVID-19 and within two weeks' time, I lost my maternal grandfather, my paternal grandfather, my uncle, and a doula colleague to COVID-19. All BIPOC individuals, all loved, all missed. Before this time, I had experienced a major loss—my father was shot and killed when I was thirteen years old—but I had never experienced so many deaths in such a short time. Even writing about this brings up raw emotions of anxiety and fear, but

---

* Chanel Porschia-Albert, "Centering a Practice of Hope to Advance Birth Justice," speech delivered at the National Perinatal Association Conference, Aurora, CO, May 3, 2022.

also physical sensations of a heavy chest and light-headedness as well as parts of my body feeling numb and disconnected. When I think about what I experience and continue to experience, I can clearly see the deep racialized trauma I experienced. COVID-19 was a racialized trauma in the ways that it was handled and the ways BIPOC bodies were deprioritized when it was obvious BIPOC communities were being affected by this the most. When COVID-19 began to impact non-BIPOC communities, changes were made to try to control the virus, but by that time, it was too late for many BIPOC individuals and communities.

I would like to pause here to say the names of the people
I have lost:

Solomon Wade III (my father)
Curtis King Sr. (my maternal grandfather)
Tracey Curtis (my uncle)
Solomon Wade Jr. (my paternal grandfather)
Angela Diaz De Leon (my doula friend)

When I began to build a relationship with my grief, I remembered the traditional stages of grief, developed by Elisabeth Kübler-Ross, that I am aware of and have also taught to my students: shock, denial, anger, bargaining, depression, and acceptance. Shock comes after moving past numbness—you are back in your body and you literally can't believe what is happening right now. Denial is a protective measure, a way of masking that shock and tucking it away because it's too hard to handle in that moment. When anger shows its face, it might be directed internally or show up externally and manifest in anger toward others. In the bargaining phase, the individual attempts to regain some control, perhaps some normalcy, over the circumstances—it is a form of desperation. After these stages are unsuccessful in managing the reality, we turn to depression, which in comparison can be a calmer and more reclusive phase. Depression moves into acceptance, which is our way of dealing with our circumstances and moving toward closure. These stages of grief did resonate with me and still do resonate with me, but it felt at the time like something was missing and not really speaking to my full lived experience of grief.

I also want to recognize that as I was experiencing loss after loss, I was also experiencing the most growth ever in my business and navigating a relationship that was close to running its course. It was also the spring and summer of 2020, a time when the many murders of unarmed Black people were being protested and spoken about on a daily basis. It felt like I was living in a kaleidoscope of racialized trauma coming in and out of my vision every minute of the day. I was holding the complexities of trying to figure out and manage my capacity to hold feelings of constant and overlapping grief, fear of death coming at any time, anger at how my Black body was proven to be continuously devalued and deprioritized, and the happiness and pride that came with seeing my businesses grow.

Being a container for all these feelings and experiences pushed me to step into my grief instead of shoving it away. I wanted to form a better relationship with my grief and literal death. In my past, I had always loved supporting birth because it felt like an honor to be at the portal of the creation of life, but now I felt the shift to experience the portal from the perspective of death. Something inevitable, but something I hadn't spent much time with. In 2021, I signed up for the Going with Grace Death Doula Training by Alua Arthur, a death doula, attorney, and adjunct professor. Being in this space of learning also encouraged my research around being in my Black body, experiencing grief, and realizing trauma healing and collective liberation are deeply connected to my healing journey and the continued healing of my community.

Death is not a medical event. It's a cultural event. It's a life event. It just is. It's not something that needs to be treated or done away with.

—Alua Arthur, founder of Going with Grace*

In my search I became aware of public health expert Stacy Scott and her perspective of Black grief using a theory developed by psychiatrist Elisabeth Kübler-Ross. As we discussed above, Kübler-Ross provides a deeper understanding of grief through five distinct stages of grief after the loss of a loved one: denial, anger, bargaining, depression, and acceptance. Scott grounds this theory by explaining that racism, such as institutional racism, has caused disproportionate Black death through crises such as COVID-19, police violence, and perinatal and infant health mortality. There are also other overlapping issues that negatively affect Black lives and create ongoing Black grief such as environmental, health, and education inequities. Due to these circumstances specific to the Black experience, Black grief is different, with ongoing generational trauma, loss, and inequities among other realities specific to Black culture. These extra layers of grief can also be true for other BIPOC communities, but I am specifically speaking to Black grief because it is my experience.

In "How Do We Address Black Grief, Compounded by Centuries of Racism, Loss and Trauma?" a blog post written by Caitlin Forbes for *Baby 1st Network*, the components of Black grief are explained in depth.

Despair

"Despair is a form of acceptance whereby a person of color understands that they may always live with the fear of underpinning loss."†

---

* Alua Arthur, "Decolonize Your Death," interview with Jumakae, *Your Story Medicine*, https://www.jumakae.com/goingwithgrace.

† Caitlin Forbes, "Blog; How Do We Address Black Grief, Compounded by Centuries of Racism, Loss, and Trauma?," *Baby 1st Network*, July 7, 2020, https://www.baby1stnetwork.org/news /blog-how-do-we-address-black-grief-compounded-centuries-racism-loss-and-trauma.

This feeling is also increased when a Black person realizes loss may be at an increased possibility simply because they are Black, not because of anything they have actually done that might lead them to experience such a high amount of loss or a high fear of loss.

I remember reading this and immediately feeling every part of my body breathe because it felt like I was finally being seen in my experience as a Black person who is consciously and subconsciously grieving at all times. Losing my loved ones caused feelings of despair, for sure, but even more so, I constantly feel the anxiety of never feeling TRULY safe. Not knowing if a underreaction of the government to a deadly virus would kill me or if going grocery shopping would be the last moments of my life, like the racially motivated shooting and murder of ten Black community members of Buffalo, New York. This awareness of despair has also made me very aware of creating safe(r) spaces for myself internally and externally, whether that is finding a space within myself that creates space for me to breathe and just be or heading to my happy place, a plant-filled meditation room in my home. Despair is highly present in my everyday life, but it does not have to become my life.

Self-Blame

"Self-blame is often a factor in coming to terms with death. But this blame can be all consuming for Black people who have spent their lives trying to keep their loved ones safe in a society that privileges the safety of White people." Black people can also hold guilt for not being able to protect themselves or others from harm, even though the factors of harm are not within their control. These uncontrollable factors can be particularly activating because they are derived from structures, systems, and people who uphold white supremacy.

This one, for me, specifically sparked a thought about power. I thought about how my Grandpa Curtis was cared for before he passed in the ICU. Soon after his death, I often thought about whether I could have been more present in some way, like could I have traveled to Philadelphia and physically been there or asked more questions to make sure he was getting the best care possible. I think about how my Blackness wouldn't have given me additional power in this hospital space, and I think about how his Blackness could have also hindered the care he received. I'm not sure, and I can't prove his Blackness affected his treatment, but it was something about not feeling like I even had enough power to get a closer look at his care or demand more, especially in the beginning of a pandemic. I didn't necessarily blame myself for his death, but there was a level of blame that felt present because the system and structures that exist do not prioritize my voice, his health, and our existence.

Move to Action

"Having the time to grieve and process loss is a privilege that is often not afforded Black people." Processing grief involves being able to feel, rest, and recover over a period of time, but many Black people are not afforded this luxury. Along with loss comes the responsibility of still maintaining their livelihood while also aiming to figure out the financial weight of burial procedures, arranging family care, and other responsibilities, ultimately delaying the grieving process for long periods of time and at other times making it impossible to grieve.

After experiencing the four deaths of BIPOC people I loved and admired to COVID-19, I really didn't get to rest or grieve in a way I would have liked. Around the time these deaths occurred, my businesses began to surge in growth—a blessing in many ways, but I didn't have the support or ability to put anything down to tend to myself. The truth is I needed the money and support coming in to *at least* bring in some financial security in a time when many of my loved ones were losing their jobs and questioning their ability to keep their necessary resources. I had to push forward for myself and for my community so I could be a possible resource for anyone needing support. Two years later, I am still fighting for my ability to do less, rest more, and grieve more. As a Black queer nonbinary woman doing this work and aiming for collective liberation despite the racism and other isms that are ingrained in my reality, there is *always* work to do. I have had to understand that rest is something I have to inject into my life no matter what may have to pause, so when I'm in action, it's coming from a place that has been allowed to grieve, to fight, and to find joy.

Endurance

"Often, Black people must find the power to endure without outside support." The mourning process intensifies after the funeral process is complete and there is now less to do and more to feel. However, for many Black people, the mask of strength that is necessary to push forward with their lives also creates an inability for others to see their vulnerability and the ways they may need to be truly supported.

In the midst of being in a time of such great loss, I remember so much still being demanded of me. Not intentionally aiming to overwhelm me or to be harmful, others were not always aware of how much was being asked of me, especially because of my Black and femme-presenting exterior. My team needed direction as we grew. My partner at the time was having her own emotional challenges and couldn't provide me with emotional support, which often left me feeling like I was in a pressure cooker 24/7. My students wanted more education and more coping skills. My family needed emotional support. The demands for my energy or time did not decrease, and there were many nights I went to bed with my chest aching. It felt like my endurance was being expanded and tested and my cries for help weren't noticed, or if they were, they weren't prioritized because I was a strong Black woman.

Survival

"For Black people, survival can be considered the new acceptance stage. If they are to survive in a system stacked against them, they have no choice but to pull themselves together and continue to persevere." The grind never stops for Black people, who are usually juggling code-switching in work spaces, financial inequities, and racism on a frequent basis along with their own relationships and care for themselves. Ongoing hardships interfere with the grieving process and can create feelings of anger, sadness, and resentment without a healthy outlet to process these feelings.

I've been blessed to work with a Black therapist whom I love and appreciate because she has supported me through the things I have shared in this book, as well as more that I'll bring to light eventually. When I began to work with her, it was a couple months out from experiencing these losses, and I specifically remember speaking with her about grief. I had guilt around not crying often and not seeming externally sad for others to see. It felt like I was grieving incorrectly, and it felt like it was a part of me I had to fix. I had to do this grieving process "the right way." She promptly told me my way of grieving was right for me and fitting to my life experiences. I told her I didn't have the privilege to just fall apart, and she validated that thought because she is Black too and can understand that survival is key. She can understand that, many times, survive is the only thing I can *do* when my heart is breaking, my safety is shaking, and I'm dealing with what's in front of me as well as the systems above me that don't value me, especially when I'm a Black person grieving and unable to operate at my full capacity. This means that feelings of grief never dissipate but are present at different levels in my body every day until collective liberation becomes my existence.

Somatic Exercise: Identifying Triggers

For Black Readers

Feelings of grief are ongoing and sometimes present themselves at unexpected times. I've had moments of feeling triggered when I least expected it. The trigger could spark from an interaction with someone, and even a smell can take me back to an experience or feeling I don't enjoy. I learned this exercise over the years and would love to share it with you as a way of recognizing and moving through triggers by giving yourself permission to heal and not just survive.

1. *Notice.*
   Inhale and exhale. Notice what you feel on, in, and around your body, including the pace of your breath, your heart rate, and your body temperature.
2. *Think back to a moment of calm.*
   Think back to a recent moment when you felt most calm, safer than you may have felt in other spaces and most like your "self." For me, this space is usually when I'm home and in the spaces I have made comfortable just for me!
3. *Identify.*
   Identify when and which part of your body began experiencing disturbance or stress. For example, a smell and its associated memory could have made your stomach begin to hurt a few minutes before doing this exercise.
4. *Replay.*
   Replay the scenario from calm state to stressed state, in slow motion. Identify people, conversations, objects, or behaviors that may have made you stressed, uncomfortable, or that stand out to you as you're replaying the recent event.
5. *Tune in.*
   Tune in to your body sensations as you recall the event and slow down and notice if there is any shift

in your body, such as a sensation of tingling, tensing, warming, numbing, or cooling in your chest, arms, legs, or anywhere else in your body.

6. *Healing hands.*
   Place your hand on the area that has experienced a shift or change and breathe deeply. If it's an overall feeling, you can simply place your hands on your heart. Stay there as long as you need.

Supporting Black Grief

It is also essential and necessary for non-Black people of color and non-BIPOC people to understand the ways to support and center Black grief. Not in a hierarchical way but in a way that includes understanding the mental, physical, spiritual, and emotional impacts in Black communities because of the issues contributing to our trauma from every aspect of life, from the Black perinatal health disparities to the impact of climate change on Black neighborhoods.

Begin with acknowledging Black grief specifically. It is important to acknowledge Black grief and its through line from generation to generation. Many of the inequities faced by Black people today were also true, and many times worse, for our Black ancestors. We have learned that trauma can become a part of DNA, which means the grief we are aiming to heal is not only ours but the grief of our lineage as well.

Stop fixating on Black death. It's one thing to be informed and assist in creating more understanding and safety for Black people. It's another thing to perpetuate Black death by obsessing without action. We see this obsession in places like social media when an individual or organization begins to post about Black death, especially recordings of Black death, as a way of increasing trauma porn (usually consisting of videos of death—often Black death—allowing folks to observe others' tragedies, detached and from the safety of their own home). Before you share images, videos, or written content about Black death, evaluate your reason for wanting to post this content and what actions you plan to take in regard to this content. Also be aware of how posting this particular content could increase the trauma of Black individuals.

Trust Black people with money and other resources. Send your resources without expecting an explanation for the use of those resources. There is often a level of exposure that is expected of Black people in order to gain assistance. It's kind of like we have to prove our needs by emphasizing the ways we haven't been able to meet our own needs. In those requests for that specific kind of exposure, Black people often take on the blame instead of rightfully placing it on the broken systems keeping people from being supported while Black. Black people should not have to expose themselves in such an extreme way in order for our needs to be seen as valid. We also shouldn't have to provide exactly where or how resources are being used so someone outside of our community can verify if these uses are valid. If you want to truly assist us, understand we know how to help ourselves and utilize additional resources in a way that is led by our community.

Send funds to Black grief practitioners. Many of them are assisting their community by offering free services at the expense of their own stability. If needed, think about what type of grief practitioners come into your mind. Is it only "professional" practitioners, like therapists? Aim to decolonize your thoughts and do research on the different types of grief practitioners, such as community healers, doulas, and community spiritual leaders. Many Black people do not have access to or interest in practitioners who are deemed valid by Western medicine. However, we do have community members providing grief support services who would benefit from external resources to continue the work that is so desperately needed.

Stop fearing Black rage. There are many reasons for Black rage, some included in this book and many others not mentioned but just as important. Aim to understand Black rage and do something using your resources or privilege to support it. If you are experiencing Black rage in a personal way, do as much as you can to avoid police interaction, if possible. We have every right to be full of anger and rage without the fear of false (or overactive) alarms being rung that continue to endanger our lives more than they already are. Black grief is often ongoing anger without a safe place to experience and feel it.

Create a culturally humble grief resource list that serves Black people specifically. Many grief spaces are catered to the non-BIPOC lens and can be more harmful than helpful to Black people. For a Black person it can be difficult to practice the vulnerability needed to move through grief with a person who doesn't understand their race, culture, community, and needs. Grief is multifaceted and often inclusive of our specific life experiences based on our identities of race, sexuality, location, and more. Providing culturally humble resources creates access to Black practitioners and options for the Black person looking for support by increasing the chances of being in a space that can provide a level of safety through the presence of familiarity and the openness to learn more.

If you are an employer, promote paid mental health days and remote working whenever possible. It may or may not always be a reality you are aware of, but the physical and mental safety of Black bodies is on the line at all times. Between things like COVID-19 and police violence, many Black people often make decisions such as taking an unpaid day off or going into an office after witnessing or becoming aware of racially motivated crimes that could easily become their own reality. That means we are often choosing our jobs and financial stability over all aspects of our personal health. This shouldn't have to be a choice.

Black Grief Matters

When we think about collective liberation, we often tie it to the freedom to be our fullest and biggest selves. Black people have often had our ability to meet our basic needs taken away throughout history and current times. Collective liberation includes the ability of all people, especially BIPOC people, to be able to grieve as well as be supported and provided resources during those times of grief. Being able to grieve completes the mental sympathetic and parasympathetic processes of fight, flight, freeze, or fawn and rest and digest. Completing these cycles and mobilizing both physical and emotional selves is key to Black healing, generational healing, and communal healing across races. In order to move to a point of decreasing the Black perinatal and infant health disparities, we have to break the cycle of forcing Black people to experience the trauma and then endure the aftermath, find blame in themselves for what has happened, and jump right back into survival mode while burying the feelings and process of grief. This is also true for Black people who are not birthing people, who are moving through systems (education, criminal justice, housing, corporate America, etc.) without the ability to grieve their experiences of daily life with the resources needed and deserved. Suppressing Black grief is an act of oppression, but supporting Black grief is a step forward for everyone on the path to collective liberation.

8

A RETURN TO BIRTH

A DIFFERENT OUTCOME FOR ALL

History has shown us that courage
can be contagious, and hope
can take on a life of its own.

—Michelle Obama, remarks at Young
African Women Leaders
Forum in South Africa in 2011

N CHAPTER 1, "In the Room Where It Happens," we talked through Reena's childbirth process in a hospital system as a Black birthing parent having her first child. No aspect of her childbirth experience was unusual—from the various emotions she and her family experienced to her diagnosis of preeclampsia and her concerns. Unfortunately, even her death during childbirth has become a frequent occurrence, shown by the current disparities for Black birthing parents. However, what happened to Reena and many other Black birthing people does not have to continue to be so frequent. Throughout this book we have talked about the history and present day of Black birthing disparities, different forms of racism, the trauma we all have been exposed to because of racism, and what it means and how it looks to take on the personal responsibility of healing trauma with the goal of freeing ourselves and our communities for collective liberation.

Through these different topics, we have also created a bigger capacity for nuance in ourselves and in others, an essential piece to succeeding in our goal of collective liberation. There won't be one right answer to how to get to collective liberation, just like there won't be one right answer to decreasing and eventually eliminating Black perinatal and infant health disparities. We have to invite nuance into the discussions and plans because binary thinking is not moving the needle on saving Black lives or the lives of the BIPOC communities as a whole. If we were to put this knowledge and skill set in use, what would Reena's birth experience have the potential to look like? Could Jarrod feel equipped for fatherhood, as well as able to be present for Reena without fear of being seen as a threat to others simply because he is a Black man? Could Hilary support Reena without pushing her own birth experience onto Reena's? Could Dr. Smith see Samantha as his equal, allowing them both to truly center Reena and her unique childbirth experience? It may be hard for some of us to even imagine a world where Black birthing people are centered and prioritized, but I am here to show you that it is possible.

Before the Day

Reena is a twenty-six-year-old Black cis woman. She is pregnant with her first child and is being supported by her partner, Jarrod, and her mother, Hilary. From the beginning of the birth process (i.e., from conception), Reena has received quality, supportive health care. She has also experienced racially concordant care—not everyone, but enough people from her community with similar experiences have participated in her care that, on the day of the birth, she feels she is in a safe space and has providers to reach out to if necessary. All her medical providers are trauma informed and have done ongoing work around anti-racism while learning how to self-regulate their own emotional and trauma responses to provide her with a supportive and patient-led experience. Reena has also decided to work with a doula to provide her with education throughout her prenatal and postpartum stages, as well as to provide her with emotional support as she moves through all the feelings that come with this new phase of her life.

Jarrod is ecstatic about having his first child with Reena, but soon after the announcement he began to have concerns about knowing as much as possible about birth so he could be supportive during the birth process. As Reena's belly became more visible, he also started to have fears of being perceived as an "angry Black man" based on experiences he himself had had, as well as the experiences of other Black men in his life. He wants to be as present as possible for Reena but questions whether he will be able to speak up without causing issues. Due to these thoughts, Jarrod has joined a support group for Black fathers, and in those spaces he has been able to talk about his fears and apprehensions, and the kind of experience he is hoping to have instead. He receives advice around how to have a safe and supportive experience for Reena and for himself, and he enters the hospital room confident and excited rather than afraid. He has also learned some self-regulation skills, and the presence of a doula has helped him with learning about the birthing process, as well as how to interact in a space that isn't necessarily one he is entirely familiar with—so that he can advocate for Reena with the certainty that he will be heard.

Finding out Reena was having a child felt like the biggest gift Hilary could receive. She was more than excited to be a grandmother, but a couple of months into Reena's pregnancy, Hilary began to have night-mares and flashbacks to the traumatic birth she experienced when having Reena. Her own experience with birth was wrought with dismissive health care; lack of informed consent, trust, and support (her sister was there, but her husband could not come in because of the rules of the times); and a dangerous, life-threatening postpartum hemorrhage that was ignored by the providers and could have led to her death.

After this difficult birth experience, Hilary reached out to her physician about her trauma symptoms and received a referral to a therapist. She attended therapy weekly and maintained her own spiritual practice, working through her personal history and trauma. With this combination of healing modalities, she became better able to be present for Reena's experience, and able to differentiate it from her own. The education that she's been able to receive has helped her to feel more confident and more present for her daughter, the exact outcome she was seeking.

Samantha's work at the hospital has shifted so that her voice is listened to with more respect and confidence in her understanding of the situation. She is not so overworked and overloaded with patients that she cannot spare the time to really listen to and observe Reena. She is also using self-regulating techniques to work through her anxiety around being homeless just a few short years ago. She and Dr. Smith have both learned how to perform collaborative care, and the hospital system that they work for now has ongoing support around mental health, trauma skills, and other psychosocial aspects of care. The hospital has put into action an accountability system that teaches restorative practices, a way to learn from mistakes and fix them without being punitive in the way the system that caused Dr. Smith to retreat from his instincts was.

Reena's doula, Jessica, has studied the full-spectrum doula care model, so she believes in client-led experiences that include the mental, physical, and spiritual health of the client and their family. Jessica has gladly taken the time to provide education that includes prenatal and postnatal care, as well as lactation and any other interests that Reena and her family have expressed. She has been present in Reena's life since the first trimester and will stay with her through the child's infancy and throughout Reena's parental experience for as long as she's needed. Jessica has also created a birth plan with Reena and her family that expresses her ideal plan for her birth—a vaginal birth with the least amount of medical interventions possible—as well as options if her birth deviates from her ideal birth.

Hilary has witnessed Reena's pregnancy experience and seen how it differs from her own. She is proud of Reena for utilizing doula services, something she was not afforded at the time she was having her children. She is overall feeling more confident and ready for what may come because of the education she obtained through the doula, including understanding Reena's medical options and choices, as well as getting a clearer understanding of how everyone will work together to support and advocate for Reena during the labor and delivery process.

On the Day

Reena has been laboring for more than twenty-four hours with Jarrod, Hilary, and Jessica by her side. She is exhausted and has expressed feeling discouraged and overwhelmed with pain because she is not progressing as fast as she expected. Rather than immediately getting an epidural, Samantha offered Reena some nonmedical options for pain control, and Jessica answered any additional questions. Reena decided to sit in a hot shower for pain relief and hoped to avoid any medical interventions unless necessary. Jarrod and Hilary take turns assisting her while she walks the halls. Reena feels supported by her entire birth team, including her doula, family, and medical providers.

A couple hours later, the birth process is still moving pretty slowly. At that point, Jessica suggests taking a walk, trying to get some information on the position of the baby, and putting this information together to figure out the best next option for Reena. Dr. Smith and Samantha, the labor and delivery nurse, reassure Reena that she is a first-time mother and it's normal to have a slower birth process, and that they are there to assist her in whatever ways she finds helpful. They also make sure to explain to Reena, Hilary, and Jarrod that as long as nothing is going actively wrong or headed in a negative direction, Reena can continue following her ideal birth plan as much as medically possible. Lastly, they open the floor for any questions and listen patiently and openly to all concerns, making sure this experience is a collaborative one.

A few hours later, Reena's blood pressure reading is unusually high. Hilary becomes very nervous but remembers that Reena's experience is not hers, so she is able to calm herself enough to be present for Reena. Jarrod is highly concerned and asks Jessica, their doula, what would be some possible next steps. Jessica encourages Reena and her family to speak to the physician about their concerns and interventions that could help to decrease Reena's blood pressure and, if all goes well, keep her on track for a vaginal delivery. Dr. Smith and Samantha come into the room and explain to Reena that she is experiencing preeclampsia. Dr. Smith takes the time to explain what preeclampsia is and possible outcomes of preeclampsia if not treated appropriately. He also assures Reena and her family that he is experienced with this diagnosis and equipped to assist Reena as much as possible with her having a positive outcome, even with the unexpected diagnosis. Dr. Smith then shares possible options for dealing with preeclampsia, such as taking magnesium sulfate intravenously to help lower the blood pressure, which could also support Reena's plan to avoid having a cesarean section. The family decides to take a few minutes to discuss the options presented to them and decide magnesium sulfate is a positive and appropriate approach to dealing with Reena's high blood pressure. Nurse Samantha then comes in and explains the process of starting the magnesium sulfate intravenously and makes sure to answer any additional questions before starting the medication. Reena begins the magnesium sulfate, feeling nervous about the unexpected diagnosis and additional medical intervention but also empowered and supported by her family and medical team. Jarrod and Hilary are also feeling uncertain about what's to come next, but they are both grateful for the ability to be by Reena's side throughout this entire process.

After some time on magnesium sulfate, Reena's blood pressure begins to lower, a positive sign that gives Reena confidence in her plan to have a vaginal birth. In between contractions, she is able to rest and eat light food, which helps her to maintain her energy. Samantha comes into the room frequently to continue monitoring her patient, and she is feeling positive about the individual care she is able to give Reena. Samantha also checks in with Hilary and Jarrod to see if they have any questions or concerns, understanding that collaborative care between all parties will only benefit Reena and her baby. Dr. Smith is also monitoring Reena from afar along with his other patients, but he has made himself very accessible to Samantha in case he is needed at any time.

As Reena's labor progresses, she is dilating more and feeling happy about the progress she's making. However, her blood pressure has begun to become a concern once again. Her readings are rising, and the magnesium sulfate is beginning to lose its effectiveness in supporting her body in lowering her blood pressure. Reena begins to feel nervous and even slightly panicked. Hilary and Jarrod stand by her side, holding her hand and rubbing her back as she begins to cry and express her fear of having a cesarean section. Dr. Smith, Samantha, Reena, Jessica, Hilary, and Jarrod decide to have another conversation about possible next steps. In the process of this conversation, an epidural becomes a part of the conversation. Originally Reena wanted to avoid using an epidural because she was fearful of the epidural process and the possible risks, such as a back injury. She also feared an epidural beginning a cascade of interventions that would lead her to the operating room. Dr. Smith listens to Reena's concerns patiently, then explains to Reena that one of the benefits of having an epidural is that it can possibly assist in lowering her blood pressure. He also explains that Reena's concerns are valid, but with the current path of her labor, he believes an epidural could assist her goal of having a vaginal birth by lowering her blood pressure and giving her body the additional time it needs to deliver her child successfully. With the support of her doula and family, Reena decides that an epidural is in fact the way that she would like to go, especially if it means adding additional time to her labor process and avoiding a cesarean section. Reena is very scared of the epidural process, especially with the large needle going through her back, and she prays that there will be no other consequences of receiving an epidural. The anesthesiologist comes into the room, introduces herself, speaks to Reena about all the risk and benefits of having an epidural, and answers any questions presented to her. The anesthesiologist also welcomes her to have a support person in the room who can help her to stay in the correct position and provide emotional support during the process. Reena decides she wants Jarrod to be there during the process. During the epidural insertion, Jarrod and Reena receive step-by-step instructions about what is happening, how it's happening, and when it's happening to provide them with clarity and support during such a vulnerable time.

After receiving the epidural, Reena decides to take a nap, and Jarrod stays by her side, also going in and out of sleep. Hilary decides to head downstairs to get some lunch for herself and Jarrod as well. During this time, Nurse Samantha continues checking on Reena and changing her positioning every couple of hours to support the baby in getting in the best placement possible for delivery. During one of her checks on Reena, she asks Reena if it is OK to give her a vaginal exam, since contractions seem to be coming quite frequently on the monitor. Reena agrees to this vaginal exam and is helped into position. Although Reena is numb from the waist down, Samantha explains the process of checking her cervix and answers any questions that arise. When Samantha completes the exam, she excitedly lets Reena and her family know Reena is fully dilated, and the baby's head is very low in her pelvis, meaning it is finally time to start preparing for delivery. Jarrod, Hilary, and Reena are beyond excited about this next step since it's all they've been waiting for. Dr. Smith comes into the room to ask Reena if she has any questions about the delivery process, and he also explains what he will be doing to support her at this step in her journey. After Dr. Smith is finished talking, Samantha and other nurses begin to set up for delivery with smiles, and an unlimited amount of that joy can be felt throughout the delivery room.

Jessica turns off the bright lights in the room and puts on the music Reena finds relaxing while also filling the room with essential oils that support Reena and the environment that she's dreamed of having during the birth of her child. During this time, Jessica also talks to Reena about what to expect at this time and reminds Reena of her strength and that her only job is focusing on herself and her baby, letting the rest of her care team do the rest. The pushing process begins, and Reena is feeling excited yet very exhausted and ready to meet her baby. This process takes a couple of hours as she moves through contractions, breathing, and feelings of frustration, happiness, fear, and exhilaration. As she is pushing her baby into the world she is also feeling wrapped up in the love, security, and support everyone has put into this experience. She begins to crown, and for a moment things become still before she hears the sound of her baby's cries. Welcome to the world, Tyler.

Immediately, Tyler is placed on Reena's chest to let them both soak up the benefits of skin to skin, including reducing stress and regulating Tyler's body temperature. A couple moments later, Reena's placenta is delivered successfully, and her preference of delayed cord clamping is fulfilled by Dr. Smith. Jarrod is able to stroke the back of his brand-new son while feeling proud of his ability to be an active support to Reena during this long and challenging process. Hilary is watching from afar and in tears as she admires her daughter's strength. Dr. Smith fills Reena with words of encouragement and opens the floor to any questions she or her family may have while also explaining what will happen next, such as the plan to help reduce the size of her uterus and getting Tyler set up to latch from her breast. As explained by Dr. Smith, Samantha begins to press on Reena's abdomen to assist her uterus in clamping down to normal size, a crucial part of the immediate postpartum stage that also assists in decreasing postpartum bleeding that can be fatal if not controlled.

After a few minutes, Samantha notices that Reena's bleeding is not reducing as much as she would like, so she quickly alerts Dr. Smith, who also agrees with Samantha's concern. Dr. Smith and Samantha explain what is happening to Reena and their concerns while Samantha increases the amount of pressure and the frequency of the abdominal massages. They explain to her that it might be helpful to take a medication that would help her uterus to contract and reduce the bleeding. They also explain that the uterus contractions would be helpful, but it would be a quicker way to reduce bleeding and decrease further complications. Reena decides to take the medication, and shortly after, she feels pain from it, which she was told to expect. She is grateful for the explanation so she could understand the medication and how it will help her with her bleeding. A few minutes later, her bleeding subsides. Everyone in the room is elated with the results of the medication, especially Hilary since she had experienced the consequences of postpartum hemorrhage herself.

Samantha and Dr. Smith continue to check on Reena and her family. Jarrod is able to be skin to skin with his son and feels grateful for the ability to be fully present and helpful to Reena during Tyler's birth process without fear of being removed from the room. Hilary is able to hold her new grandson and feels tired but satisfied with the care Reena received. Reena is grateful for her experience. It may not have turned out the way that she wanted, but during the process she felt supported and as in control as she could be. She's grateful for the support of her doula, Jessica, and her family as well as her medical team, Dr. Smith, Samantha, and the other nurses in the hospital space. And, most important, Reena has not become a part of the perinatal mortality statistics and has survived a normal part of life that has unfortunately become a deadly experience for many people who look like her.

The Difference

Through collective liberation, the birthing parent, Reena, lived through her childbirth experience, and, more than that (because survival is the absolute minimum Reena should be able to expect), her birthing experience was centered around her and her needs. She received education and support throughout her pregnancy from her doula, Jessica, who was there to answer any questions and provide resources for Reena and her family. She came out on the other side of her birth feeling supported and basking in love for her child. Although she did not experience her ideal birth, her care team worked hand in hand with her and her family to come as close as possible to her personal goals of avoiding a cesarean section.

Hilary, Reena's mother, naturally worried about her daughter's safety but felt confidence in the tools and caregivers provided to Reena, such as Reena's doula and the care team's standard of explaining every step and unexpected change throughout the experience. She was also actively working on her trauma with therapy and other tools, so she was able to stay present for her daughter in the birth room and not interject into Reena's experience with her own fears and trauma.

Jarrod, Reena's partner, was able to work through his trauma around not being able to speak up without being perceived as an angry Black man, so that if or when he noticed something going awry, he would not only say so but would be listened to. He also felt the support of the community that he connected with and was able to express his fears and apprehension about being in a hospital space as a new Black father. He was able to enter into fatherhood with a feeling of belonging, presence, and love.

Nurse Samantha felt secure in her position as an experienced labor and delivery nurse and was able to voice her opinion to the doctor with the assurance that her observations and concerns would be taken into account and respected. She was able to focus on Reena and do her job in a way that was in alignment with her values rather than being overwhelmed by procedures and by the power dynamics that exist in health care today.

Dr. Smith processed his trauma around the death of his previous patient, allowing him to make decisions based on what was happening in the moment, trusting his own instincts and knowledge rather than blindly following hospital guidelines or making decisions highly influenced by his past. He was more secure in his own capabilities, which allowed him to see Reena's care as a collaborative effort rather than something that he alone was in charge of. He was a better doctor because he understood the power he obtained with his identities and education and mindfully decided to return power to the people and communities he served.

There were also systemic changes that took place in this improved version of Reena's experience that could not be obviously seen. The hospital system Reena was a patient in increased training opportunities for all employees to include ongoing education about trauma-informed care, anti-racism, inclusion, ableism, and other topics that emphasized the importance of care and respect for the many different communities the employees served. An accountability system was also created to track the positive and negative outcomes of the care provided in the hospital. This accountability system not only provided education when needed but also removed professionals if their care was not in alignment with the mission of equity for all. Professionals in the space were also educated about the history of racism and discrimination in the health care system, understanding that without awareness and action, the racial divide in health care would only continue to widen.

These are the same people, with all the same traumas and issues— but personal and systemic changes have shifted the individuals and, by default, their communities. When people are given the tools and resources needed to improve themselves, their community also becomes more resourced, more inclusive, and much healthier.

A Return to Birth

The only way to a new, improved, and safe world for all people, especially Black and Indigenous people and people of color, is to return to birth. This means returning to what birth once meant, before it was severely medicalized and industrialized. Before those happenings, birth was a process of trusting in our knowledge of our own bodies, our own experience, and our own practices. There was concrete information that was important to study and practice for the safety of birthing people, but there was also the knowing of birthing people. Their physical and emotional intuition led the experience that belonged to them and only them, instead of the current power dynamics present in birth spaces that take the power of birth away from birthing people and place it into the hands of those who have not received the holistic education needed to create healthy communities, healthy parents, and healthy babies.

Our return to birth must first be a community effort, including all BIPOC and non-BIPOC people, meaning no one is left behind and only stakeholders in their respective communities are seen as the leaders of this process. A return to birth must be conducted with great purpose and unrelenting passion and strength, for as we return to birth, we return to ourselves, our communities, and the literal life of the beings that will be born in the future. If we can make this new world the standard, our babies will become adults who only operate with these goals and ways of existing in mind.

Next steps for many individuals will be to start their commitment to personal trauma healing by understanding their identities, their role in our current world, and what experiences or traumas may contribute to their life in a way that can no longer continue. It means recognizing the ways you may have committed harm but also the ways that your existence has been a blessing to others. Recognize how your life may need to slow down, shift, and even pause as you do this deep, ongoing work to create healing opportunities for yourself and your community. The work is internal more than external. If we want to create change by deconstructing systems and innovating ways to exist that have not been created yet, we have to start within. It's going to get ugly. It's also going to be cathartic. Even more important, it's necessary for a continued healthier experience.

Communities will need to come together with internal and external stakeholders to have conversations about their histories and answer important questions such as: Who was this community built for? What is the history of leadership in this community? What is needed in this community, and why haven't those needs been met before? What is the future of this community, and what will it take to get there? There is no doubt that these questions will bring up disruptions and feelings of grief. Things often have to get messy and picked apart for us to understand how we got to where we are and where we need to go. These necessary conversations can also move the community into a space of innovation, making sure that its members are creating the path to a healthier community with necessary resources and support, and that people of privilege are utilizing that privilege to make it happen. In order for things to change, these actions have to begin.

To sustain this return to birth, non-BIPOC communities must maintain the shift of shared power to BIPOC communities and continue to build the capacity for cultural differences. Hierarchical practices must be condemned, and community-based, patient-led experiences have to become the standard. Most important, a return to birth means we all have to continuously commit to doing the self-work of liberation. Although this work is sometimes unbelievably hard and earth shattering, we must understand that our liberation is intrinsically connected to that of every human being on this earth.

Birth Neoterism

As a next step to collective liberation, I want to introduce you into a new framework I have built to pull all the context of this book into a structure that is clear, comprehensive, and action oriented. I am inviting you to become a *birth neoterist*, a person who is forward focused and dedicated to innovation and sustainability for creating a pathway to a new reality for birth. I am welcoming you into a space that goes beyond statistics and into using the knowledge of ancestors and ourselves to push change and, more important, positive impact for birthing people.

As birth neoterists, we understand the reproductive justice framework as the foundation and the path to collective liberation, and we utilize history as a way of supporting forward-focused thinking and creation for the future of birth. We support the full spectrum of reproductive experiences and the variation of people having those experiences. We prioritize an ongoing personal trauma healing practice for the well-being of ourselves and our community. We also design and implement innovative and sustainable systems to create a better future for all birthing people. We value people, knowledge, healing, equity, and innovation because all these pieces are vital on the path of creating structures and reimagined systems that will impact both birthing and nonbirthing people of all identities.

Somatic Exercise: Feeling a New World

For All Readers

At this point, you have learned and felt so much throughout this book. Now it is time not only to see the future but also to feel it in your body. Before beginning this exercise, find a comfortable place and bring a notebook with you.

1. Get into a comfortable position. Begin taking deep, cleansing breaths, imagining your breath coming through the top of your head and releasing through the bottom of your feet. Take as many breaths as necessary until you feel you have created enough space within yourself to invite creativity.
2. In your notebook or in this book, write out some thoughts related to this book that excite you. For example, building a healthy community can spark a feeling of excitement throughout your body. Take a few more breaths, inviting expansive thoughts based on what excites you in the moment.
3. Next, write down any ideas that come to mind for the future of birth. Don't put any pressure on yourself to

have a plan. You can also use the following questions
to prompt your thoughts.

   a. What resources do you wish existed for yourself?
What have others in your community wished for?

   b. What tools and resources do you feel would
be beneficial to birth workers (doulas, doctors,
nurses, etc.)? Is it a new technology? Is it a specific education?

   c. Are there systems that you would like to exist outside of our current systems? What is needed to
start the process of creation?

   d. What do you feel like needs to be eliminated alto-
gether? What could replace it?

4. When you finish writing out your expansive thoughts,
close your eyes and sit with them. What physical
sensations are you experiencing? What emotions are
you feeling? How does it feel to dream and create
the future? Write any additional notes down and plan
to do this exercise often. This practice can lead to
idea generation, creative plans, and, most important,
action forward for the improved future we all need.

We can no longer wait for birthing people to be centered; instead, we move this initiative forward ourselves, with or without support from the systems that have created this reality. We can no longer continue to repeat mortality statistics of Black and Indigenous communities without action. It is time to mobilize, to innovate, and to move forward. It is time to return to birth in order to build the future of birth. It is time for the wisdom of BIPOC communities to be valued and prioritized, and for the privilege and knowledge of non-BIPOC communities to move us forward. This is the work we must do together, aware of our humanity while holding nuance, because we and future generations deserve less despair and more intergenerational hope.

You are not free until I am free.

RESOURCE LIST

People and Organizations

Kimberly Seals Aller, who created the Irth (Birth Without Bias) App, an app for Black and Brown people to leave reviews on perinatal and pediatric health care providers.
https://irthapp.com/

Ancient Song Doula Services, founded by Chanel Porschia, with the aim of providing high-quality, holistic doula care to people of color regardless of ability to pay.
https://www.ancientsongdoulaservices.com/

Alua Arthur, death doula, recovering attorney, and the founder of Going with Grace providing end of life (death doula) training.
https://goingwithgrace.com/

Black Mamas ATX, governed by the Black Mama Community Collective founded by Dr. Michele Rountree.
https://blackmamasatx.com/

Stephanie Brown, IBCLC, of Nourish and Nurture Lactation, an inclusive lactation wellness provider.
https://www.nnlactation.com/

Rachel Cargle, writer, entrepreneur, philanthropic innovator.
https://rachelcargle.com/

Commonsense Childbirth School of Midwifery, founded by Jennie Joseph, providing safe and equitable midwifery care, and training others to do the same.
https://commonsensechildbirth.org/

Dr. Joy Cooper, cofounder of Culture Care, a platform for connecting with culturally aligned physicians.
https://www.ourculturecare.com/

Jarrah Foster, IBCLC, founder of Lactation & Wellness, an inclusive lactation wellness provider.
https://www.lactwell.com/

Amber Rose Isaac, a New York mother who died during childbirth. Save a Rose Foundation is a nonprofit started in her honor that seeks to eliminate flaws in the health system that contribute to the perinatal health crisis.
https://www.savearosefoundation.org/

Charlie Johnson, founder of 4Kira4Moms, an organization aiming to increase awareness and education around the human rights issue of perinatal mortality.
https://4kira4moms.com/

Ibram X. Kendi, author, historian, anti-racist scholar, and recipient of the MacArthur Fellowship.
https://www.ibramxkendi.com/

Rachael Lorenzo (Mescalero Apache / Laguna Pueblo / Xicana), who started Indigenous Women Rising (IWRising), an organization aiming to increase awareness and access to health care for Indigenous communities.
https://www.iwrising.org/

Resmaa Menakem, anti-racist educator.
https://www.resmaa.com/

Stephanie Mitchell, midwife and owner of Birth Sanctuary Gainesville, the first freestanding, Black-owned birth center in Alabama.
https://thebirthsanctuary.com/

Nurturely, a nonprofit based in Eugene, Oregon, created by Ayesha Elliot, that offers the Milk Mood Moves conference and the program Nurturing BLACK: Baby's Lived Experience as Cultural Kinship.
https://nurturely.org/

Ocama Collective, a Toronto-based group of community-directed birth workers of color, dedicated to the reclamation of traditional and holistic childbearing and birthing practices among queer and trans IBPOC folx.
https://www.ocamacollective.com/

Postpartum Healing Lodge, founded by Raeanne Madison, services and online training for birth workers who serve Indigenous communities.
https://postpartumhealinglodge.com/

Brittany Packnett Cunningham, activist, educator, writer, leader at the intersection of culture and justice.
https://brittanypacknett.com/

Cristen Pascucci, founder of Birth Monopoly, an organization mapping obstetric violence and bringing the ownership of birth back to the individual.
https://birthmonopoly.com/

Dr. Karen A. Scott, associate professor of OB-GYN and reproductive sciences.
https://www.birthingculturalrigor.com/

SisterSong, a southern based reproductive justice advocacy group.
https://www.sistersong.net/

Breonna Taylor, a Black woman shot and murdered in her home by police. Stand with Bre is a Grassroots Law Project to raise support, action, and awareness.
https://www.standwithbre.com/

Cheyenne Varner, founder of The Educated Birth, a platform for inclusive content, imagery, and representation in birth and reproductive health.
https://www.theeducatedbirth.com/

Books

The Big Letdown: How Medicine, Big Business, and Feminism Undermine Breastfeeding by Kimberly Seals Aller
The Boy Who Was Raised as a Dog by Bruce Perry

The First-Time Parent's Childbirth Handbook: A Step-by-Step Guide for Building Your Birth Plan by Stephanie Mitchell

It Didn't Start with You by Mark Wolynn

Motherwit, an Alabama Midwife's Story by Onnie Lee Logan

Pushout: The Criminalization of Black Girls in Schools by Monique Morris

Reproductive Justice: An Introduction by Loretta Ross and Rickie Solinger

Skimmed: Breastfeeding, Race, and Injustice by Andrea Freeman

BIBLIOGRAPHY

Agency for Health Care Research and Quality. "Executive Summary." 2019 National Healthcare Quality and Disparities Report. Published December 2020. https://www.ahrq.gov/sites/default/files/wysiwyg/research/findings/nhqrdr/2019qdr.pdf.

Aron, Nina Renata. "Meet the Unheralded Women Who Saved Mothers' Lives and Delivered Babies Before Modern Medicine." *Timeline.* January 11, 2018. https://timeline.com/granny-midwives-birthed-rural-babies-and-saved-lives-33f12601ba84.

Arthur, Alua. "Decolonize Your Death." Interview with Jumakae. *Your Story Medicine.* https://www.jumakae.com/goingwithgrace.

Austin, Beth. "1619: Virginia's First Africans." Hampton History Museum: Make History with Us. December 31, 2019. https://hampton.gov/DocumentCenter/View/24075/1619-Virginias-First-Africans?bidId=.

Baldwin, James. "As Much Truth as One Can Bear." New York Times Book Review, *New York Times*, January 14, 1962.

Bartlett, Jessica, "Internal Analysis Shows Black Patients at Brigham Faced More Security Calls." *The Boston Globe.* May 23, 2022. https://www.bostonglobe.com/2022/05/23/metro/black-patients-brigham-womens-are-nearly-twice-likely-have-security-called-them-white-patients/.

Birth Monopoly. "Obstetric Violence." Accessed June 15, 2022. https://birthmonopoly.com/obstetric-violence/.

Carpenter, Zoë. "What's Killing America's Black Infants? Racism is Fueling a National Health Crisis." *Nation*. February 15, 2017. https://www.thenation .com/article/archive/whats-killing-americas-black-infants/.

Centers for Disease Control and Prevention. "Breastfeeding Disparities Exist." Breastfeeding Facts. Accessed June 15, 2022. https://www.cdc.gov/breastfeeding /data/facts.html.

Centers for Disease Control and Prevention. "Causes of Infant Mortality." Infant Mortality. Accessed June 15, 2022. https://www.cdc.gov/reproductivehealth /maternalinfanthealth/infantmortality.htm.

Charles Smith, Margaret, and Linda J. Holes. *Listen to Me Good: The Story of an Alabama Midwife*. Columbus, OH: Ohio State University Press, 1996.

Children's Hospital. "What You Need to Know About SIDS." Sudden Infant Death Syndrome (SIDS). Accessed June 15, 2022. https://www.childrenshospital .org/conditions/sudden-infant-death-syndrome-sids.

Coleman-Jensen, Alisha, Matthew P. Rabbit, Christian A. Gregory, and Anita Singh. "Household Food Security in the United States in 2020." US Department of Agriculture. Economic Research Report Number 298. https://www .ers.usda.gov/webdocs/publications/102076/err-298.pdf?v=7786.

Cooper, Joy. "Racially-Concordant Care: Why It Matters if Your Provider Looks Like You." For Families (blog), Hi Cleo, February 1, 2021. https://hicleo.com /resource/racially-concordant-care-why-it-matters-if-your-provider-looks -like-you/.

Covert, Bryce. "Too Often, a New Baby Brings Big Debt." *The Nation*, May 15, 2012. https://www.thenation.com/article/archive/too-often-new-baby-brings -big-debt/.

Dane County Health Council. "Dane County Health Council and Partners Announce Black Maternal and Child Health Alliance to Lead Local Birth Equity Efforts." *University of Wisconsin-Madison News*, September 18, 2020. https://news.wisc.edu/dane-county-health-council-and-partners-announce -historic-launch-of-the-black-maternal-and-child-health-alliance-to-lead -local-birth-equity-efforts/.

Davis, Angela. "UCLA Red Lays Ouster Proceedings to Racism." Interview with Ken Reich. *LA Times*, September 24, 1969. https://latimesblogs.latimes.com /thedailymirror/2009/09/ucla-fires-angela-davis.html.

Department of Labor. "Frequently Asked Questions and Answers About the Revisions to the Family and Medical Leave Act." Wage and Hour Division. DOL.

Accessed June 15, 2022. https://www.dol.gov/agencies/whd/fmla/final-rule
/faq.

Department of Labor. "Section 7(r) of the Fair Labor Standards Act—Break Time
for Nursing Mothers Provision." Wage and Hour Division. DOL. Accessed
June 15, 2022. https://www.dol.gov/agencies/whd/nursing-mothers/law.

Department of Labor. "Fact Sheet #73: Break Time for Nursing Mothers under the
FSLA." Wage and Hour Division. DOL. Accessed June 15, 2022. https://www
.dol.gov/agencies/whd/fact-sheets/73-flsa-break-time-nursing-mothers.

Dethmer, Jim. "The Cognitive Emotive Loop: What It Is, Why It Keeps You Stuck,
and How to Break Free." Conscious Leadership Group. March 21, 2018.
https://conscious.is/blogs/the-cognitive-emotive-loop-what-it-is-why-it
-keeps-you-stuck-and-how-to-break-free.

DiAngelo, Robin. "Ziet Campus Transcript." Accessed June 15, 2022. https://
robindiangelo.com/wp-content/uploads/2018/08/zeit-campus-transcript
.pdf.

Dill, Janette, Odichinma Akosionu, J'Mag Karbeah, and Carrie Henning-Smith.
"Addressing Systemic Racial Inequity in the Health Care Workforce." *Health
Affairs*, September 10, 2020. https://www.healthaffairs.org/do/10.1377
/forefront.20200908.133196.

"Facts: Racial Economic Inequality." *Inequality.org*. Accessed June 15, 2022.
https://inequality.org/facts/racial-inequality/.

FitzGerald, Chloë, and Samia Hurst. "Implicit Bias in Healthcare Professionals:
A Systematic Review." *BMC Medical Ethics* 18, no. 1 (2017): 19. doi: 10.1186
/s12910-017-0179-8.

Forbes, Caitlin. "Blog; How Do We Address Black Grief, Compounded by Centuries of Racism, Loss, and Trauma?" *Baby 1st Network*. July 7, 2020. https://
www.baby1stnetwork.org/news/blog-how-do-we-address-black-grief
-compounded-centuries-racism-loss-and-trauma.

Freeman, Andrea. "From Breastfeeding to Beyoncé, 'Skimmed' Tells a New
Story About Black Motherhood." Interview by Breandrea July. *Public Health*, NPR, February 11, 2020. https://www.npr.org/sections/health
-shots/2020/02/11/801343800/from-breastfeeding-to-beyonc-skimmed
-tells-a-new-story-about-black-motherhood.

Freeman, Andrea. *Skimmed: Breastfeeding, Race, and Injustice*. Stanford, CA:
Stanford University Press, 2020.

Geronimus, Arline T., Margaret Hicken, Danya Keene, and John Bound. "'Weathering' and Age Patterns of Allostatic Load Scores Among Blacks and Whites in the United States." *American Journal of Public Health* 96, no. 5 (May 2006): 826–833.

Gillespie, Claire. "How Systemic Racism Contributes to Less Breastfeeding Amongst Black Mothers." Family and Parenting News, *Very Well Family*, February 24, 2021. https://www.verywellfamily.com/why-are-black-women-less-likely-to-breastfeed-5113076.

Giorou, Evangelina, Maria Skokou, Stuart P. Andrew, Konstantina Alexopoulou, Philippos Gourzis, and Eleni Kelastopulu. "Complex Posttraumatic Stress disorder: The Need to Consolidate a Distinctual Syndrome or to Reevaluate Features of Psychiatric Disorders Following Interpersonal Trauma?" *World Journal of Psychology* 8, no. 1 (March 2018): 12–19. doi: 10.5498/wjp.v8.i1.12.

Greenwood, Brad N., Rachel R. Hardeman, Laura Huang, and Aaron Sojourner. "Physician-Patient Racial Concordance and Disparities in Birthing Mortality for Newborns." *Proceedings of the National Academies of Sciences of the United States of America* 117, no. 35 (2020): 21194–21200. doi: 10.1073/pnas.1913405117.

Hasa. "Difference Between PTSD and Complex PTSD." Pediaa. Accessed June 15, 2022. https://pediaa.com/difference-between-ptsd-and-complex-ptsd/.

Indigenous Women Rising. "About Indigenous Women Rising." accessed June 15, 2022, https://www.iwrising.org/about-iwr.

Infographics. "Infographic: 6 Guiding Principles to a Trauma-Informed Approach." CDC. Accessed June 15, 2022. https://www.cdc.gov/cpr/infographics/6_principles_trauma_info.htm.

Johnson, Charles. "Black Mothers Matter: Racism and Childbirth in America." BBM Panel. *Hollywood Health and Society*, May 21, 2019. Audio, 37:34. https://youtu.be/DVi46ErwY00.

Kirti, Kamna. "The Tragic Plight of Enslaved Wet Nurses: How Black Mothers Were Systematically Deprived of Breastfeeding Their Own Children." *Lessons from History*, Medium. August 2, 2020. https://medium.com/lessons-from-history/the-tragic-plight-of-enslaved-wet-nurses-b1c80b73f290.

Lawrence, Elizabeth. "What Doctors Aren't Always Taught: How to Spot Racism in Health Care." *KHN*. November 17, 2020. https://khn.org/news/racism-in-health-care-what-medical-schools-teach/.

Lee, Hedwig, Michael Esposito, Frank Edwards, Yung Chun, and Michal Grinstein-Weiss. "The Demographics of Racial Inequality in the United States." Brookings. July 27, 2020. https://www.brookings.edu/blog/up -front/2020/07/27/the-demographics-of-racial-inequality-in-the-united -states/.

"Life Story: Anarcha, Betsy, and Lucy: The Mothers of Modern Gynecology: The Story of Enslaved Women Who Were Forced to Undergo Experimental Surgeries That Laid the Foundations for Modern Gynecology." *Women and the American Story.* https://wams.nyhistory.org/a-nation-divided/antebellum /anarcha-betsy-lucy/#resource.

Logan, Onnie Lee, and Katherine Clark. *Motherwit: An Alabama Midwife's Story.* Belmont, CA: Untreed Reads Publishing, 2014.

McIntyre III, Bruce. "New York Mother Dies After Raising Alarm on Hospital Neglect." Interview by Alexandra Villarreal. *The Guardian*, May 2, 2020. https:// www.theguardian.com/us-news/2020/may/02/amber-rose-isaac-new-york -childbirth-death.

Medical Association of the State of Alabama. "Racial Disparities." Save Alabama Moms. Accessed June 15, 2022. https://alabamamedicine.org /savealmoms/#1574279800496-da6debc5-5990.

Menakem, Resmaa. *My Grandmother's Hands: Racialized Trauma and the Pathway to Mending Our Hearts and Bodies.* Las Vegas: Central Recovery Press, 2017.

Merriam-Webster. "Trauma." *Merriam-Webster.* Accessed June 15, 2022. https:// www.merriam-webster.com/dictionary/trauma.

Mitchell, Stephanie (@doctor_midwife). "Getting Right to the RJ shits w/ @doctor _midwife." Instagram live @sabia_wade, filmed April 18, 2022. https://www .instagram.com/p/CcgHyuKJuav/.

"Milk, Mood, Moves." Continuing Professional Development. School of Medicine at Oregon Health and Science University. accessed June 15, 2022. https:// www.ohsu.edu/school-of-medicine/cpd/milk-mood-moves.

Morris, Monique W. *Pushout: The Criminalization of Black Girls in Schools.* New York: The New Press, 2015.

National Academies of Sciences, Engineering, and Medicine. *Birth Settings in America: Outcomes, Quality, Access, and Choice.* Washington, DC: The National Academies Press, 2020. https://doi.org/10.17226/25636.

Niven, Steven J. "Motherwit: Onnie Lee Logans 4 Decades as a Midwife in Ala." *The Root*, March 28, 2016. https://www.theroot.com/motherwit-onnie-lee -logan-s-4-decades-as-a-midwife-in-1790854770.

Obama, Michelle. "Remarks by the First Lady During Keynote Address at Young Adult Women Leaders Forum." South Africa, The White House: President Barack Obama. June 22, 2011. https://obamawhitehouse.archives.gov/the -press-office/2011/06/22/remarks-first-lady-during-keynote-address -young-african-women-leaders-fo.

Ocama Collective. "Mission." Accessed June 15, 2022. https://www.ocamacollective .com/about.

Owens, Deirdre Cooper, and Sharla M. Fett. "Black Maternal and Infant Health: Historical Legacies of Slavery." *American Journal of Public Health* 109, no. 10 (October 2019): 1342–1345. doi: 10.2105/AJPH.2019.305243.

Perry, Bruce, and Maia Szalavitz. *The Boy Who Was Raised as a Dog: And Other Stories from a Child Psychiatrist's Notebook: What Traumatized Children Can Teach Us About Loss, Love, and Healing.* New York: Basic Books, 2007.

Porschia-Albert, Chanel. "Centering a Practice of Hope to Advance Birth Justice." Speech Delivered at the National Perinatal Association Conference, Aurora, CO, May 3, 2022.

Rayburn, William F., Imam M. Xierali, Laura Castillo-Page, and Mark A. Nivet. "Racial and Ethnic Differences Between Obstetrician-Gynecologists and Other Adult Medical Specialists." *Obstetrics and Gynecology* 127, no 1. (2016): 148–152. doi:10.1097/AOG.0000000000001184.

Roberts, Dorothy. *Killing the Black Body: Race Reproduction and the Meaning of Liberty.* New York: Vintage Books, 1997.

SAMHSA's Trauma and Justice Strategic Initiative. "SAMHSA's Concept of Trauma and Guidance for a Trauma-Informed Approach." Substance Abuse and Mental Health Services Administration. June 2014. https://store.samhsa.gov /sites/default/files/d7/priv/sma14-4884.pdf.

Sartin, Jeffrey S. "J. Marion Sims, the Father of Gynecology: Hero or Villain?" *Southern Medical Journal* 97, no. 5. (2004): 500–505. doi:10.1097/00007611 -200405000-00017.

Schellpfeffer, Michael A, Kate H. Gillespie, Angela M. Rohan, and Sarah P. Black- well. "A Review of Pregnancy-Related Maternal Mortality in Wisconsin, 2006–2010." *Wisconsin Medical Journal* 114, no. 5 (2015): 202–207.

"School-to-Prison Pipeline." ACLU: American Civil Liberties Union. Accessed June 15, 2022. https://www.aclu.org/issues/juvenile-justice/school-prison-pipeline/school-prison-pipeline-infographic.

Scott King, Coretta. "King's Widow Urges Acts of Compassion." *LA Times.* Transcript of speech delivered at service summit, January 2000. https://www.latimes.com/archives/la-xpm-2000-jan-17-mn-54832-story.html.

Scott, Karen. "Black Mothers Matter: Racism and Childbirth in America." BBM Panel. *Hollywood Health and Society*, May 21, 2019. Audio, 38:56. https://youtu.be/DVi46ErwY00.

Shen, Megan Johnson, Emily B. Peterson , Rosario Costas-Muñiz, Migda Hunter Hernandez, Sarah T. Jewell, Konstantina Matsoukas, and Carma L. Bylund. "The Effects of Race and Racial Concordance on Patient-Physician Communication: A Systematic Review of the Literature." *Journal of Racial and Ethnic Health Disparities* 5, no. 1 (2018): 117–140. doi: 10.1007/s40615-017-0350-4.

SisterSong. "To Achieve Reproductive Justice, We Must . . ." Reproductive Justice. SisterSong: Women of Color Reproductive Justice Collective. Accessed June 15, 2022. https://www.sistersong.net/reproductive-justice.

Spurlock, John. "Vesicovaginal Fistula." *Medscape.* November 11, 2021. https://emedicine.medscape.com/article/267943-overview.

Susan B. Anthony Collection. *Narrative of Sojourner Truth; A Bondswoman of Olden Time, Emancipated by the New York Legislature in the Early Part of the Present Century; with a History of Her Labors and Correspondence Drawn from Her "Book of Life."* Battle Creek, MI, 1878. https://www.loc.gov/item/29025244/.

Taylor, Alison M., Jo Alexander, Edwin van Teijlingen, and Kath M. Ryan. "Commercialisation and Commodification of Breastfeeding: Video Diaries by First-Time Mothers." *International Breastfeeding Journal* 15, no. 33 (2020): 1–11. https://doi.org/10.1186/s13006-020-00264-1.

Taylor, Sonya Renee. *The Body Is Not an Apology: The Power of Radical Self-Love.* Oakland, CA: Berrett-Koehler Publishers, 2021.

Thompson, John, Kawai Tanabe, Rachel Moon, Edwin Mitchell, Cliona Mcgarvey, David Tappin, Peter Sidebotham, and Fern Hauck. "Duration of Breastfeeding and Risk of SIDS: An Individual Participant Data Meta-Analysis." *Pediatrics* 140 (2017). doi: 10.1542/peds.2017-1324.

Valtis, Yannis K., Kristen E. Stevenson, Emily M. Murphy, Jennifer Y. Hong, Moshin Ali, Sejal Shah, Adrienne Taylor, Karthik Sivashanker, and Evan M.

Shannon. "Race and Ethnicity and the Utilization of Security Responses in a Hospital Setting." *Journal of General Internal Medicine* (2022). https://doi .org/10.1007/s11606-022-07525-1.

Vennemann, M., T. Bajanowski, B. Brinkmann, G. Jorch, K. Yücesan, C. Sauer-land, and E. Mitchell. "Does Breastfeeding Reduce the Risk of Sudden Infant Death Syndrome?" *Pediatrics* 123, no. 3 (2009): 406–10. doi: 10.1542.

Vollers, Anna Claire. "Midwives Can Legally Deliver Alabama Babies for First Time in Decades as State Issues Licenses." *AL*, January 19, 2019. https://www .al.com/news/2019/01/midwives-can-legally-deliver-alabama-babies-for -first-time-in-decades-as-state-issues-licenses.html.

Wall, L. Lewis. "The Medical Ethics of Dr. J. Marion Sims: A Fresh Look at the His-torical Record." *Journal of Medical Ethics* 32, no. 6 (2006): 346–350. https:// doi.org/10.1136/jme.2005.012559.

Walls, Bryan. "Freedom Marker: Courage and Creativity." *Underground Railroad: The William Still Story*, PBS. Accessed June 15, 2022. https://www.pbs.org /black-culture/shows/list/underground-railroad/stories-freedom/henry -box-brown/.

"What Is a Peer?" MHA: Mental Health America. Accessed June 15, 2022. https:// www.mhanational.org/what-peer.

"What Is Posttraumatic Stress Disorder (PTSD)?" American Psychiatric Associa-tion. Accessed June 15, 2022. https://www.psychiatry.org/patients-families /ptsd/what-is-ptsd.

Williams, Janiya M. "Disrupting Disparities & Exclusion in Lactation." National Committee for Responsive Philanthropy. September 16, 2021. https://www .ncrp.org/2021/09/disrupting-lactation-disparities.html#.

Wolynn, Mark. *It Didn't Start with You: How Inherited Family Trauma Shapes Who We Are and How to End the Cycle.* New York: Viking, 2016.

Your Fat Friend. "The Bizarre and Racist History of the BMI." Elemental. October 15, 2019. https://elemental.medium.com/the-bizarre-and-racist-history-of -the-bmi-7d8dc2aa33bb.

Yurkanin, Amy. "Why Do Black Women Get More Hysterectomies in the South?" Center for Health Journalism. February 1, 2022. https://center forhealthjournalism.org/2022/01/28/why-do-black-women-get-more -hysterectomies-south.